The Guinea Pig Club in Numbers

The Guinea Pig Club in Numbers

Archibald McIndoe and Reconstructing Injured Aircrew in WW2

Colin Pateman

FRONTLINE BOOKS

First published in Great Britain in 2026 by
Frontline Books
An imprint of Pen & Sword Books Limited
Yorkshire – Philadelphia

ISBN 978 1 03619 018 7

A CIP catalogue record for this book is available from the British Library.

Typeset by Mac Style
Printed in the UK by CPI Group (UK) Ltd, Croydon, CR0 4YY.

FSC www.fsc.org
MIX
Paper | Supporting responsible forestry
FSC® C013604

The Publisher's authorised representative in the EU for product safety is Authorised Rep Compliance Ltd., Ground Floor, 71 Lower Baggot Street, Dublin D02 P593, Ireland.
www.arccompliance.com

For a complete list of Pen & Sword titles please contact:

PEN & SWORD BOOKS LIMITED
47 Church Street, Barnsley, South Yorkshire, S70 2AS, England
E-mail: enquiries@pen-and-sword.co.uk
Website: www.pen-and-sword.co.uk
or
PEN AND SWORD BOOKS
1950 Lawrence Road, Havertown, PA 19083, USA
E-mail: uspen-and-sword@casematepublishers.com
Website: www.penandswordbooks.com

Contents

Introduction

During the Second World War, the Queen Victoria Cottage Hospital at East Grinstead was an 'Emergency Medical Services Scheme Hospital'. It was not a Royal Air Force Hospital, and therefore was not staffed by Princess Mary's Royal Air Force Nursing Service personnel. This precluded the hospital from compiling forms F540, Operational Record Books which were required to be completed at all Royal Air Force Hospitals. This creates an anomaly, because the Queen Victoria Hospital in East Grinstead was consistently occupied by RAF and Commonwealth Air Force pilot and air crew patients. It was a nominated hospital by the emergency scheme for airmen and pilots, in particular burn victims, to receive treatment. The hospital operated at full capacity for the majority of the war years. In addition, once built, the separate Canadian Wing for Canadian aviators also operated at high capacity until the end of the war. Much of this success rests with the management across the hospital by plastic surgeon Archibald McIndoe and his medical team.

The absence of F540 forms denies many aspects of post-war research and investigations, in particular to the history of The Guinea Pig Club. It was a unique club which evolved and developed at the hospital by the seriously burnt and injured Battle of Britain pilots in 1940 and 1941, all of whom were under the supervision of Archibald McIndoe.

The Guinea Pig Club has now become steeped in RAF history. It holds a historical position in having responsibly educated the general public during the war years, in particular the residents of East Grinstead, but more widespread by newspaper reporting and the reporting by war correspondents. Archibald McIndoe had the vision to run an impeccable surgical facility within a hospital ward that was far removed from the normal hospital infrastructures at that time. He did so when the country was in great peril from Nazi Germany, spearheaded by Luftwaffe aircraft which significantly outnumbered the aircraft of the RAF.

The Guinea Pig Club initially had a most restricted membership criteria created by the Battle of Britain pilots, men who had endured terrifying fires in their cockpits. Thereafter, the club was impacted by the strategic bombing campaign which greatly influenced later membership. These matters were fundamental in establishing the number of honoured men who became McIndoe's Guinea Pigs. However, it is now impossible to quote that definitive membership with certainty. The club lives on in history today, carrying the accepted membership total of **649**. The late Bob Marchant, the last custodian of the Guinea Pig Club membership secretary, and the last person who had worked alongside McIndoe, always adhered to the previously quoted membership figure. It is of benefit to know that Archibald McIndoe frequently made mention that the club had a membership of over **600**. It appears he never uttered a definitive number of patients who became his 'Guinea Pigs'.

The first known published roll of membership by Edward Bishop was in 1963. This provides a membership total of **635**. *The Guinea Pig Club* (Macmillan and Co, St Martin's Press).

The second published roll in 1979 by Peter Williams and Ted Harrison provides a figure of **642**. *McIndoe's Army* (Pelham Books).

The Guinea Pig Club memorial board displayed at the Queen Victoria Hospital, erected in the year 2000, displayed **643** names.

The third published roll in 2002, again by Edward Bishop, provides a figure of **643**. *McIndoe's Army* (Grubb Street).

Emily Mayhew in 2004 provides a reference to the club's membership as **647**. *The Reconstruction of Warriors* (Greenhill Books).

The author adds that despite the original restrictive criteria of membership created in 1941, Archibald McIndoe freely accepted and operated upon personnel from other services who were not pilots or aircrew. Flying had been a primary requisite to joining the Guinea Pig Club, but McIndoe often personally selected patients. By example, John Hills was amongst **18** people admitted to hospital after an aircraft crashed and spewed burning aviation fuel amongst the ground crew. He suffered deep burn injuries to his hands, face and legs. McIndoe admitted him into the Queen Victoria Hospital from Cosford Hospital. He was surrounded by pilots and aircrew who accepted him without reservation. His reconstructive surgery of twenty operations and becoming a member of the Guinea Pig Club changed his life. It was McIndoe who chose John to act as his driver in the immediate post-war

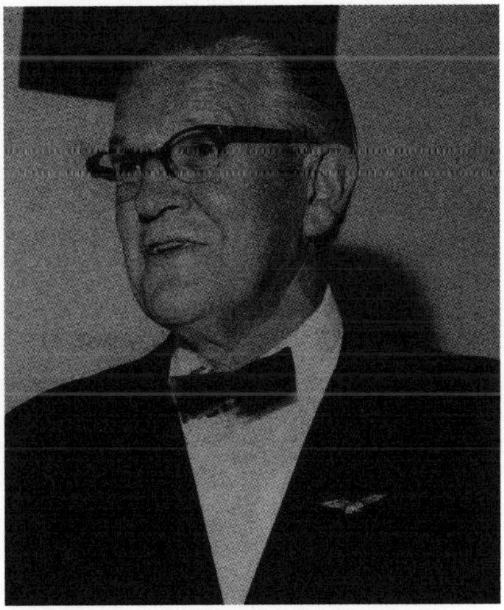

Sir Archibald McIndoe seen wearing the Guinea Pig Club badge. He maintained lifelong friendships with some of the Guinea Pigs. He continued to operate on club members who needed medical assistance long after the war, whilst he managed a successful private practice in plastic surgery.

period. Other patients from differing military services and civilians were also treated by McIndoe and his medical teams. Some in absence of being airmen are recorded as members of the Guinea Pig Club, either erroneously or otherwise. Notably a few airmen who are indisputably Guinea Pigs, are not duly recorded in detail.

The Guinea Pig Club in Numbers will provide an understanding of many of the patients who joined this special club. It also divulges facts and statistics which are unexpected, interesting and revealing in many aspects. It was unlike the Goldfish Club for airmen shot down into the sea who survived by a rubber dinghy and the Caterpillar Club, men who saved their lives by parachute. Those men were required to officially apply to join those associations. No official application process was required for becoming a Guinea Pig, the definition of which was a club working in the interests of disabled Air Force men of all Allied Nations who have been, or are, patients at The Queen Victoria Hospital.

The Hospital's collection of records, patient files, drawings and photographs that document the work of Archibald McIndoe are now held at the West Sussex Record Office in Chichester. A Wellcome Trust grant has allowed the documents to be catalogued and preserved. The archive and selected records have been preserved in partnership with the Guinea Pig Club and East Grinstead Museum. The author has researched and collated information upon the Guinea Pig Club over several years. He is indebted to the late Bob Marchant for access to the museum's archives. McIndoe's legacy is today carried forward in the Blond McIndoe Foundation, founded in 1961.

Colin Pateman, 2026

Chapter 1

The Founding of Friendships Amongst Guinea Pig Patients

1 Leading Aircraftsman William Cruickshank could arguably be recognised as the first airman to become a Guinea Pig. He is also amongst the youngest of the Guinea Pigs, being just **19** years of age. Tragedy and bad luck struck under most questionable circumstances for him on 28 October 1939. He was an air gunner on board an Avro Anson, conducting convoy protection duties. That day, three Spitfires sighted the convoy and adopted an attack position as they closed on the Anson, assuming it to be an enemy aircraft. One Spitfire fired its guns, raking the Anson's fuselage, before the aircraft was identified as friendly. Bill Cruickshank was struck, gunfire ripping into his jaw shattering it. The Anson's wings, tail, fuel tank and undercarriage were all damaged. The Anson crew fired recognition flares upon which the Spitfires departed. Landing at Leuchars the jaw injuries inflicted upon Bill Cruickshank were most apparent, with all the associated horror that it had been inflicted by mistaken identity. The subsequent enquiry exposed that the Spitfire pilots were not aware that convoys were being protected by Royal Air Force aircraft. Nineteen-year-old Bill Cruickshank arrived at the Queen Victoria Hospital on 2 November 1939. It appears he was to become Guinea Pig number one. The need for jaw reconstruction involved **6** complex operations for Archibald McIndoe.[1]

58 The origin of the Guinea Pig Club rests with the events which took place during the Battle of Britain in 1940. Fighter pilots primarily in Hurricane and Spitfire aircraft defended England from the German military forces who were intent on a potential invasion of the British Isles. However, another influence, the British Commonwealth Air Training Plan signed in Canada on 17 December 1939, by the governments of the United Kingdom, Canada, Australia, and New Zealand, also significantly impacted upon the Guinea Pig Club membership. Canada created **58** flying schools. These were safe environments where it was hoped to train and create substantial

numbers of aircrews. The target of airmen to be trained was ambitious at **520** pilots with basic flying capability, and **544** pilots with advance flying capability, **340** observers and **580** wireless operator-air gunners every month. Nearly **2,000** trainee aircrew personnel per month would flow into an operational training structure in the United Kingdom. This unsurprisingly created significant numbers of training casualties many of whom suffered serious burns and facial injuries whilst preparing for operational flying against the enemy.

13

Medical Officer Squadron Leader Rexford-Welch quoted that by the end of April 1940, only **13** non-fatal burn casualties had been recorded. However, by midsummer the service had encountered many severe burns to significant parts, namely the face and hands and in July 1940, the RAF consultants in surgery and the civilian consultant in plastic surgery Archibald McIndoe formed a sub-committee on burns. This signalled the cessation of the treatment of burn cases as general surgical patients in general wards, where they were liable to cross-infection from general surgical cases. They would come under the care of teams of surgical personnel trained in plastic surgical principles of early skin coverage and healing by skin grafts. The Air Ministry instituted an efficient method of notifying burn casualties to a Central Medical Establishment so that consultants and surgical specialists of the RAF could rapidly visit aircrew casualties in civil hospitals.[2]

1

Reputedly **1** unknown RAF pilot was waiting for an appointment at the operating theatre at the Queen Victoria Hospital when he wryly remarked, 'What a life – we're nothing but a plastic-surgeon's guinea pig'. This could well have been the comment which led to the name of the club which was gradually coming into being at the hospital. During the winter of 1940 and into 1941, skin grafts and saline baths induced long periods of recovery for many burnt airmen. This created a spirit of togetherness through pain and discomfort and it brought a great camaraderie and became known as the 'Spirit of Ward Three'.[3] Little imagination is required to appreciate the pain, discomfort and mental anguish that each patient endured.

20

South African Guinea Pig, Walter Godfrey Courteney Edmonds from Cape Town, underwent **20** operations at the Queen Victoria Hospital. Archibald McIndoe is known to have suggested his injuries were amongst the worst he had attended to. Walter had sustained deep burn injuries on 4 March 1940 following a crash whilst training at Upper Hayford in Oxfordshire. Shortly after a night take-off, he lost control of the Hampden aircraft which crashed, bursting into flames. The hospital at Halton transferred Edmonds into the care of McIndoe on 1 April 1940. His surgery was significant, eyelids, ears and facial repair. It was almost six years later when Edmonds eventually departed England, returning home to Cape Town in December 1945.[4]

34 There were **34** Guinea Pig Club members who fought in the Battle of Britain between 10 July 1940 – 31 October 1940.[5] **544** airmen were killed in the Battle of Britain, amongst them were **6** aircrew who were just **18** years of age. One was Laurie Rasmussen, the youngest New Zealander to take part in the Battle of Britain, killed in a flying accident on 4 September 1940.[6]

15 The Battle of Britain reached its climax on **15** September 1940. The Luftwaffe launched a relentless assault in the skies over Britain. It was a day of heavy fighting, and the Luftwaffe suffered significant casualties and a decisive defeat. The costly raid finally convinced the German high command that the Luftwaffe could not achieve air supremacy over Britain, a vital requirement for the invasion of the British Isles. For this reason, that date is accepted and celebrated as Battle of Britain Day. However, aerial combat continued with fierce ferocity over the British Isles. The founder members of the Guinea Pig Club, and the many which followed all recognise this pivotal and important period of conflict.

15 Roy McGowan was shot down during the climatical dogfights that occurred on **15** September 1940. It was during an enemy interception over the North Weald to Kent area when he was attacked by the enemy fighters whilst engaging their bombers. Roy McGowan's Hurricane was on fire and he parachuted out landing in the Thames Estuary. He spent about **30** minutes in the water, before being picked up from the Kent side of the Thames. Flying Officer McGowan suffered from burns to his face, hands and legs as well as shrapnel injuries to his leg and left ankle. He was taken to the Hospital in Rochester before being transferred to Basingstoke and onward to East Grinstead on 6 December 1940. The number of operations he had to endure at the Queen Victoria Hospital is unknown. This Battle of Britain Guinea Pig successfully returned to operational flying and survived the war.[7]

3

The Guinea Pig Club originated from patients all of whom had received surgery and the skills of care from the **3** doctors McIndoe, Hunter and Mullins. It is accepted that this evolution took place in July 1941. Those summer days would lead to a most exclusive club being formed. Those injured men considered themselves the Guinea Pigs for the expert surgery undertaken by Archibald McIndoe and his medical team. Membership rules to join the club evolved, but always required the necessity to have been operated upon by McIndoe himself.[8] The allegiance to McIndoe amongst the Guinea Pigs was unwavering and it was likewise respected by him. The small group of burn injury patients had no idea this club would become embedded in the history of the RAF.

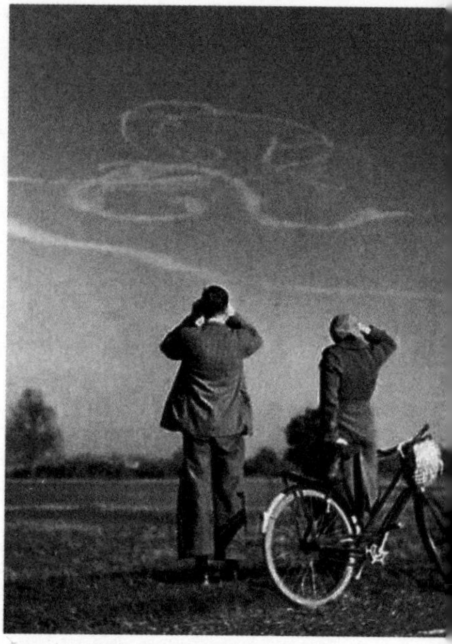

Vapour trails were observed in the skies over southern England during the Battle of Britain. These trails, formed by the condensation of water vapour in the exhaust of aircraft in dogfights between British and German planes.

7

The formation of the club led to **7** men creating a committee. They were Archibald McIndoe, Tom Gleave, Peter Weeks, Geoff Page, Russell Davies, Michael Coote and Bill Towers-Perkins. The now immortalised black humour amongst the injured men rose to the fore when Flying Officer Towers-Perkins was appointed as the very first club secretary. It was assumed that his injuries were such that it was impossible for him to write. Pilot Officer Weeks was appointed as the first treasurer for the club. He was unable to walk, thereby assuring that the funds would not disappear. The club president was appointed as Archibald McIndoe, and Vice President was Squadron Leader Tom Gleave, proudly wearing his new nose constructed for him by McIndoe. The new skin was grown by Gleave himself when McIndoe created a tube pedicle. The movement of tube pedicles from one part of the patient to an adjacent area was known as 'waltzing'. As the tube pedicle was moved up the body, it took **3** weeks for the blood supply to establish itself after each movement. This meant the airmen had to get used to holding themselves in

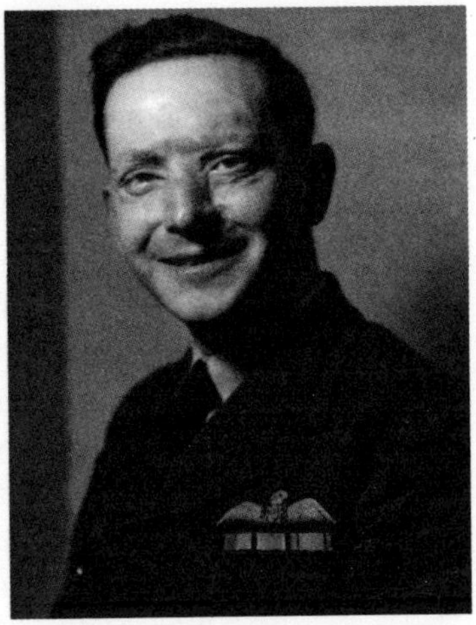

Flying Officer Towers-Perkins was appointed as the founding Guinea Pig Club secretary. He had been wounded on 1 September 1940, successfully parachuting out of his Hurricane having suffered burns after aerial combat with a Luftwaffe bomber near to Tunbridge Wells. He had landed no more than **15** miles distant from the Queen Victoria Hospital. He was admitted to the Kent & Sussex Hospital, Tunbridge Wells and moved on 4 November into the care of Archibald McIndoe. His burn injuries required surgery over the next **2** years. He is seen wearing his pilot's tunic and the trio of medal ribbons. Interestingly, the rosette indicating the award of The Battle of Britain Bar to his 1939-1945 campaign star is absent.

awkward positions with restricted movement. Although devised by Harold Gillies, McIndoe developed the process ensuring that unburnt tissue from distant sites was used to reconstruct and replace burnt tissues. It was a system which was used to recreate airmen's noses, foreheads, lips, chin or facial features.

2/6

During the formation of the Guinea Pig Club, the rules stated that the club must meet once a year. Club members attending were primarily RAF personnel, generally fighter pilots including Polish and Czech airmen. The names were registered and recorded by Geoff Page. The Guinea Pig Club notes recorded by Geoff Page disclose that the club's objectives were to promote good fellowship among its members and to maintain contact with the Queen Victoria Hospital. All members were required to pay an annual subscription of two shillings and six pence, **2/6**d.[9]

19

Research indicates that **19** members initially enrolled into the Guinea Pig Club.

15

15 of the **19** members are identified by family names – Lock, Hillary, Fleming, Lord, Hart, Bennions, Truhlar, Koukal, Noble, Mann, Krasnodebski, McPhail, Banham, Smith-Barry and Butcher. These members are positively identified as:

> Reginald Lord suffered burn injuries to his face and hands after his Wellington bomber had crashed into trees on 2 September 1940 in Norfolk. He had arrived at East Grinstead hospital for treatment the following month.

Brian Noble had escaped from his Hurricane aircraft by parachute over Biggin Hill on 1 September 1940. He had his injuries treated at Sevenoaks Hospital before his delayed arrival at East Grinstead.

Richard Hillary also suffered burn injuries to his hands face and legs inflicted on 3 September 1940. He had escaped by parachute into the English Channel and was rescued by lifeboat. His recovery commenced after admission into East Grinstead Hospital, **2** months after he sustained his injuries. McIndoe achieved significant improvements to Hillary's hands in 1941 but his dexterity was much impaired.

Josef Koukal was a Czechoslovak and a fighter pilot. He had been shot down and parachuted out over the Isle of Sheppey on 7 September 1940. Koukal was receiving treatment for his burn injuries sustained after his cockpit was engulfed in flames when his fuel tank was hit. Josef Koukal occupied the bed next to Tom Gleave in Ward Three and endured **28** surgical operations for his injuries.[10] Mrs Carrie Wright, the wife of the farmer who had extinguished the flames on Koukal's clothes when he had landed by parachute, visited Josef on numerous occasions during his **2** years of hospital treatment.

Zdzislaw Krasnodebski had been shot down on 6 September 1940. This was the day prior to his Czechoslovak Ward Three comrade Josef Koukal. Krasnodebski parachuted out from his Hurricane, badly burned. The Hurricane crashed on Langley Park Golf Course near Beckenham, Kent. He was admitted to Farnborough Hospital and later transferred to the Queen Victoria Hospital, East Grinstead to be treated for his burns. In December 1940 General Sikorski, the commander of the Allied Polish forces, personally presented the Virtuti Militari medal to him.

John Fleming was shot down in flames over Tunbridge Wells on 8 September 1940. He experienced a parachute escape at great height and was found badly burnt. He was taken to a local hospital before being transferred to the Royal Air Force Hospital Halton, where he refused a double leg amputation. When John Fleming eventually arrived in Ward Three, he was placed three beds away from Frantisek Truhlar. Fleming was eventually able to return to serve but not as a pilot.

Frantisek Truhlar from Czechoslovakia was flying in a Wellington bomber on 16 October 1940. Returning from occupied Europe with a damaged aircraft, the crew flew into a balloon barrage. They crashed close to Bentley Priory near Stanmore and the bomber burst into flames. Frantisek Truhlar was later admitted to the Queen Victoria Hospital in East Grinstead, severely burned and frostbitten. His treatment enabled his gradual recovery. In post-war Czechoslovakia, when flying over his native town on his birthday, 3 December 1946, he lost his life when he crashed into a rooftop.

James MacPhail, a Spitfire pilot, parachuted out from his aircraft on 23 September 1940. He sustained burn injuries to his hands and face and like many of the casualties in 1940 he was transferred between hospitals before arriving at the Queen Victoria Hospital for treatment on 8 October. His treatment was such that he was able to return to flying duties in 1941. Most fortunately James survived the war despite a second emergency parachute escape whilst ferrying a Spitfire to Hawkinge.

George Bennions had sustained burn injuries to his face and the right side of his body when he was shot down in his Spitfire over Sussex on 1 October 1940. Having escaped by parachute, he suffered head and facial wounds including blindness in one eye, injuries which restricted his subsequent return to combat flying duties. George Bennions had shot down several enemy aircraft, and was awarded the Distinguished Flying Cross, which was announced on the day he sustained the burn injuries over the Sussex landscape.

Arthur Banham was shot down in flames in his Hurricane over Kent on 15 October 1940. His face and hands were burned during his escape by parachute and within **5** days he was receiving treatment by Archibald McIndoe. This was his second emergency parachute escape and remarkably he returned to active flying duty over Malta and Italy in 1943.

Jack Mann was shot down in March 1941, crash landing with burn injuries. The Distinguished Flying Medal recommendation awarded to him indicates he had been required to force land on **5** previous occasions. The last incident saw him resident as a patient at East Grinstead for **5** months.

Robert Smith-Barry, deemed an elderly pilot at the age of 54, had been undertaking aircraft ferrying duties. On 16 October 1940, he crashed in a Blenheim light bomber. He sustained facial injuries with serious fractures arriving at the East Grinstead hospital on 1 November 1940. Smith-Barry had flown in the 1914–18 war on nighttime anti-Zeppelin patrols.[11]

Eric Lock, a most successful Spitfire pilot, was shot down on 17 November 1940. He managed a forced landing but a serious arm injury prevented him from getting out of the cockpit. He was eventually helped out and was eternally grateful that his aircraft never caught fire. It was his arm injury that required the attention of Archibald McIndoe, as did both of his legs. Many operations were required over **6** months to remove the penetrating splinters in his legs.

Paul Hart had been flying a training aircraft when it crashed into the Welsh countryside. He arrived in East Grinstead on 23 December 1940 with significant facial injuries and endured over **20** reconstructive facial operations.

Derek Butcher crashed in a Sunderland flying boat and suffered significant injuries with his scalp torn and one eye hanging from its socket. The rescue boat crew assumed he was dead. He was revived and arrived at East Grinstead on 15 March 1941. He remained in hospital for a year before returning to flying duties as an instructor. Derek Butcher changed his name to Derek Dudley Martin in 1949.[12]

4

4 names from the **19** listed as members – Harrison, Dewar, Shephard and Langdale have not been positively identified. It is with some certainty that they were not airmen who flew in the Battle of Britain. These relatively common family names prohibit further research.[13]

8

8 names from the initial **19** listed members of the Guinea Pig Club had saved their lives by parachute.

2

The Battle of Britain fighter pilots primarily flew in **2** aircraft, the Spitfire and Hurricane. The Spitfire had two fuel tanks, one above the other behind the instrument panel in front of the pilot. The top tank held **48** gallons and the bottom tank **37** gallons. The Hurricane had **33**-gallon tanks in the wings, one on each side of the centre section, and a reserve tank behind the instrument panel holding **28** gallons. When a wing tank in the Hurricane caught fire, flames would sweep towards the reserve tank and thereafter into the pilot's cockpit.

1

The Battle of Britain Hurricane pilot Thomas Gleave was shot down on 31 August 1940, suffering burn injuries. He had witnessed Squadron Leader Harold Starr who flew with him the previous day taking to his parachute. Suspended below his parachute and floating downwards

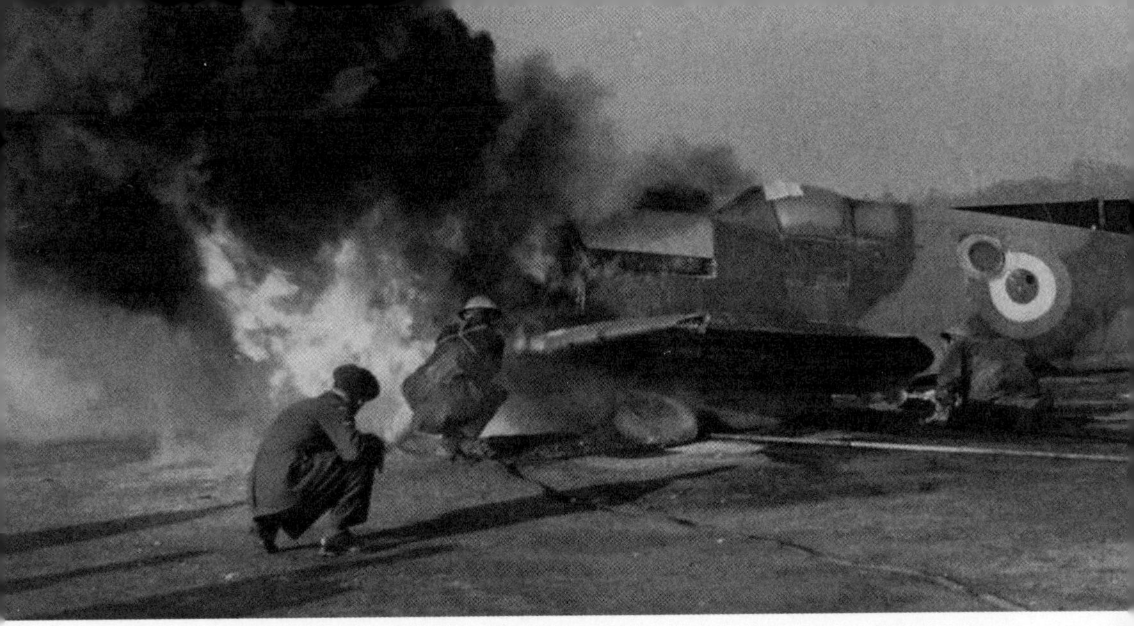

Spitfire force-landed with defective undercarriage, the ensuing fire from the ruptured fuel system starting to engulf the aircraft.

a trio of Luftwaffe fighters rounded on the helpless Starr. Below him, Mr H. Bennett, a gardener, witnessed the machine-gunning which killed him. He stated 'I saw a parachute coming down over the Hammill Brickworks. As most of the dog-fights took place at some altitude, I didn't hear or see the aircraft, but as the parachute came drifting down, I saw quite a number of enemy aircraft circling. Suddenly one of the Messerschmitts dived towards the pilot on the parachute, and then the rest also piled in. I could hear the sound of machine gunning.' A local newspaper reported his death under the title 'Victim of Nazi Barbarity' and confirmed his death as only the second occasion of which such underhand tactics had been known to have been employed by the enemy. Thomas Gleave's parachute escape was relatively uneventful. He was taken to Orpington Hospital for initial treatment before he arrived at the East Grinstead Hospital on 29 October 1940. Thereafter, Gleave became a most significant Guinea Pig and later represented the entire membership of the club as their Chief Guinea Pig in the years to come.[14]

14

One of the most unfortunate and incorrect attributions to being a Guinea Pig relates to Robert Francis Thomas Doe, a man who is regarded as one of the most successful fighter pilots of the Battle of Britain, with **14** victories. He achieved those victories flying both the Spitfire and Hurricane fighter aircraft. He joined the Caterpillar Club when he was shot down on 10 October 1940. Having parachuted out safely, he landed on Brownsea Island Dorset. He was wounded in the shoulder and leg but had avoided any burn injuries. His Hurricane crashed into the ground near Corfe Castle. Doe was taken to Poole

Hospital and recovered in time to rejoin his squadron at the end of December. On 3 January 1941, he was flying on a night patrol over the sea and above cloud, when his aircraft's oil cooler became frozen. Descending towards Warmwell, Dorset, the engine stopped completely and he made a high-speed glide approach, known as a dead-stick landing. The force of landing resulted in his harness breaking and he was thrown forward, breaking an arm and severely damaging his face on the gunsight. His nose was displaced and it is at this point that he is declared as becoming a member of the Guinea Pig Club. Robert Doe was actually taken to Park Prewett hospital near Basingstoke. The plastic surgeon Sir Harold Gillies did much of his work at Park Prewett. Gillies was assisted at Park Prewett by the surgeon J. B. Cuthbert. It was Gillies, the distant cousin of Archibald McIndoe who operated upon Robert Doe, therefore he was not a Guinea Pig despite the many published accounts stating him as being so.[15]

4

Inflicted burn injuries often contributed to by the displacement of **4** items worn by the pilots, their goggles, oxygen masks, gloves and flying jacket. Facial burns were less severe if a mask and helmet remained in place, but a total head burn often occurred when these items were torn away when escaping from a flaming cockpit.

114

In 1940, burn injuries to airmen which were confined to the neck and facial areas, amounted to **114**.[16]

120

In 1940 burn injuries to airmen upon their hands arms and upper arms amounted to **120**.[17]

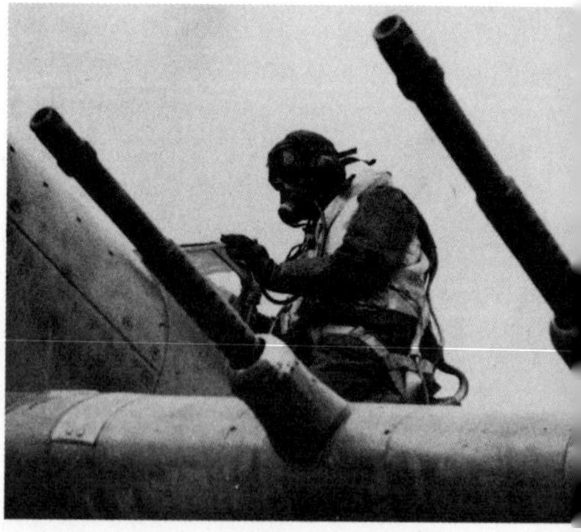

A Fighter Command pilot climbing into his cockpit wearing the full protection of gloves, mask and goggles.

1

As far as is known, only **1** Guinea Pig formally wrote to Irvin Air Chutes in Letchworth using the Queen Victoria Hospital's official letter headed paper. This occurred on 2 May 1941, when Squadron Leader Thomas Gleave wrote. 'On August 31 1940, I escaped by parachute from a Hurricane aircraft after being set on fire by enemy action. I was wearing an Irvin seat type parachute at the time. I am very keen to possess one of the Caterpillar Badges which, I believe, you present to new members of the "Caterpillar Club". Would you therefore consider this request for a badge. I enclose herewith a chit from the Station Kenley confirming my descent by parachute. I regret not having applied at an earlier date but I have since been under treatment for burns received on that date. Thanking you, yours faithfully.'

The Group Captain at RAF Kenley confirmed the facts and that the parachute used by Thomas Gleave had been manufactured by Irvin. This was a prerequisite to issuing an engraved Caterpillar Pin through written confirmation of the facts.[18]

2 Sergeant George Stroud parachuted from his burning Hurricane on 5 December 1940. He landed not far from the town of Rye in Sussex. He was taken to Rye Cottage Hospital for treatment before transportation to East Grinstead. George Stroud is attributed as having shot down 2 enemy aircraft the 1st in the Battle of Britain as well as the 2nd an Italian Fiat G.50 Freccia fighter aircraft whist flying in the Western Desert campaign in 1942. George in his later years wore both his Caterpillar Club and Guinea Pig badge at every opportunity. His daughter wore both badges proudly at his funeral in 1998.[19]

1 The most decorated Polish Battle of Britain Guinea Pig pilot was Zdzisław Krasnodebski. Awarded the Polish Silver Cross of the War Order of Virtuti Militari, the Polish Cross of Valour, and the Air Medal four times, he also received the British 1939-1945 Star with Battle of Britain clasp, Air Crew Europe Star, Defence Medal and War Medal 1939-1945.

5 George Philippi, a pilot who had been shot down and wounded in France in 1916, rose to the rank of Wing-Commander in the Second World War. He was responsible for the admission of fellow First World War pilot Robert Smith-Barry into East Grinstead Hospital in 1940. Philippi volunteered to act together with Smith-Barry as Liaison Officers between the hospital and the Air Ministry with which he was well connected. This pair of elderly pilots worked together to support the resettlement and habitation for the early Guinea Pigs and they were fundamental in delivering the Ministry of Labour scheme P5 for resettlement of disabled persons at the Air Ministry Headquarters, in Adastral House London. Archibald McIndoe was forever grateful that they extensively assisted with civil employment

structures for his Guinea Pigs. In 1950, Archibald McIndoe publicly announced the Guinea Pig Club's pleasure in acknowledging the debt owed to Wing Commander Philippi.[20]

90 The Air Ministry ruled that airmen would be discharged if they were unable to return to duty within **90** days of injury. Archibald McIndoe estimated patients with severe burns needed on average between **10** and **50** surgeries, requiring up to **3** years of treatment. The **90**-day requirement was completely inappropriate to the injuries sustained by his patients and he successfully fought to have the Air Ministry regulation removed.

1 Stanley Calton from the Royal Air Force Medical Branch was posted to the Queen Victoria Hospital to ensure that records for all service personnel were maintained, additionally ensuring that personal funds were available to each patient. Archibald McIndoe saw this as being of utmost importance for their independence and social activity within the town of East Grinstead.[21]

30 Archibald McIndoe influenced and challenged authority to such levels that Parliament extended paid convalescence for Royal Air Force crew injuries for **30** months. Additionally, McIndoe secured his patients' rights to continue wearing their uniforms. Moreover, and significantly the pay for airmen continued until the last medical intervention which was normally the final surgical operation before they were discharged from service.

649 The number of men who are regarded as having been members of the Guinea Pig Club. The East Grinstead Museum data base identifies where known, the nationality of each patient.[22]

312 The Guinea Pig Club contingent of men identified as British nationality.

3 Within the British contingent of Guinea Pigs serving in the RAF there are **3** individuals identified as Medical Officers. H. Spooner, C. R. Jenkins[23] and R. G. Chitham.[24]

4 According to the known data there were **4** individuals serving in the RAF Regiment who joined the Guinea Pig Club. Their names upon the Roll of Honour are identified as Charles Briggs, Robert Charles, John Jones and Arthur McConnell. These men were ground-based soldiers.

3 **3** British men are recorded as patients who had been serving within the British Army. They are Archibald Ball of the Royal Army Ordnance Corps, John Scott of the Black Watch Regiment and John Thompson who served in an unidentified unit.

42 The club contingent of Australians.

15 The club contingent of patients from New Zealand.

62 The number of Guinea Pigs without an identified nationality.

155 The club contingent identified as of Canadian nationality.

11 **11** men are identified as American. In all probability these will have flown as volunteers within the Royal Canadian Air Force. This number, and others not diligently recorded enhanced the Canadian nationality statistic towards the often quoted **176** Canadian Guinea Pigs.[25]

1 One individual of Canadian nationality is recorded with a status of Civilian who was treated for medical causes not connected to military service. This is an unexplained anomaly.

12 The club contingent of South African nationality.

16 The club contingent of Polish nationality.

7 The French contingent of Guinea Pigs.

5 The Czech nationality was represented with **5** patients.

2 The Dutch and Turkish nationality were represented equally with a pair each.

1 The club contingent having one member each were Russia, Greece, Argentina,[26] Egypt and Belgium.

0 Zero available records of membership. By example, the American volunteer who flew with the Royal Canadian Air Force Frederick Holbrook Mahn. He endured **18** months in the Queen Victoria Hospital and both legs were amputated below the knee in May 1943. This Guinea Pig Club member is not listed on the 'Roll of Honour board.' The author assumes his death from other causes on 5 March 1946 may explain this situation. The Canadian John Phillip Calder also provides evidence where an error exists on the Guinea Pig Club 'Roll of Honour board'. Jack, as he was known, had the misfortune of parachuting out with his crew over neutral Ireland on 24 October 1941. He was placed in a secure camp until being released on 8 July 1943. He returned to flying duties only to be involved in a crash whilst training in an Anson aircraft at night on 9 August 1943. The aircraft struck Green Gable Hill in Scotland. He sustained a fractured jaw, loss of teeth, head lacerations and a damaged left knee. Two of the crew were killed, and only good fortune saw him eventually rescued by inquisitive hill walkers. After initial care, Jack was admitted to the Queen Victoria Hospital on 13 August 1943. Jack was a former Canadian press writer, and he corresponded from East Grinstead with a newspaper account of his 'Finest surgery care at the plastic surgery and jaw injury center at the Queen Victoria Hospital'. It was published in Canada with his article supported by a photograph of him in uniform. Jack Calder left the hospital after **7** months of care and resumed flying as a navigator on Mosquito aircraft. On 20 July 1944, he and his pilot were shot down returning from an operation at Hamburg. Both parachuted away but Jack drowned in the Elbe Estuary. His body was found **6** weeks later by German fishermen at Brunsbuttel. His pilot survived to become a prisoner of war.[27] Once again, the author assumes his death in 1944 may explain the absence of his record as having been a member of the Guinea Pig Club.

0 Berrington-Pickett is a name within the register of Guinea Pigs for which the register has no detail. The author has established that a Harvard being flown by a student pilot and instructor on 18 January 1940 hit trees and crashed near Chipping Norton in Oxfordshire. The South African instructor was Pilot Officer Noel Eric Berrington-Pickett who survived. It is the author's perception that this was this incident that identifies this man.[28]

193 The number of identified Guinea Pig Club members who were serving as pilots.

27 The number of identified Guinea Pig fighter pilots who flew the Supermarine Spitfire.[29]

25 The number of identified Guinea Pig fighter pilots who flew the Hawker Hurricane.[30]

52 The number of identified Guinea Pig Club members who were crew in Wellington bombers.[31]

30 The number of identified Guinea Pig Club members who were crew in Lancaster heavy bombers.

28 The number of identified Guinea Pig Club members who were crew in Halifax heavy bombers.

61 The number of identified Air Gunners who became Guinea Pigs.

56 The number of Navigator/Observers who became Guinea Pigs.

6 The small number of men who became Guinea Pigs whilst serving as Flight Engineers.

41 The number of men who flew as Wireless Operators/Air Gunners.

11 The number of identified Bomb Aimers who became Guinea Pigs.

41 The number of Guinea Pigs who were captured and became prisoners of war.

281 Unknown trades of service personnel who are recorded within the membership of the club.[32]

1 Russell Davies was one of the founding anaesthetists at the Queen Victoria Hospital, becoming a significant member of Archibald McIndoe's surgery operating team. Also appointed as the medical officer to the club, Davies provided medical and pastoral care to the

Guinea Pigs. He would eventually assume the position as head of the anaesthesia team at East Grinstead and pioneered the development of an effective surgical recovery unit there.[33]

1 George Morley of the RAF medical branch, joined McIndoe's surgical team in the autumn of 1940. In 1941 he was appointed to the burns centre at Ely where he served until 1945. He rose to the rank of Air Vice-Marshal [34]

1 Bill Gardner was **1** of only **2** identified civilians to receive medical surgery and resident hospital care amongst the Guinea Pig Club patients in Ward Three of the Queen Victoria Hospital. As a civilian committee member to the club, he was a most popular and well-regarded person. The first edition of the club's newsletter in 1944 paid a tribute to his care and compassion to all of the Guinea Pigs.[35] His operation to remove his teeth took place in early 1949.[36]

2 The second civilian is poorly registered and simply identified as A. J. Lord. A **54**-year-old Canadian suffering from a tumour which was operated upon on 11 March 1944. For the registration of this member, it has to be presumed there was an unknown military service connection.[37]

1 One man of importance to the Guinea Pigs was Edward Blacksell. He followed in the footsteps of George Philippi and Smith-Barry providing welfare and rehabilitation services. Blacksell was always addressed as 'Blackie' and recognised for his kindness. He had enlisted in the RAF in December 1940. He became a physical training instructor and after gaining general experience was posted to the Queen Victoria Hospital in February 1943. He arrived as the Guinea Pig Club itself grew in its sense of purpose. Archibald McIndoe utilised Edward Blacksell to support the welfare and rehabilitation of the Guinea Pigs. Together, Blackie and McIndoe delivered welfare care to their patients with great devotion to duty and deploying highly creative methods Blackie became very adept in rebuilding morale. He served on the hospital Welfare Committee and liaised with the Red Cross, the Air Ministry Rehabilitation Dept and the Guinea Pig Club committee to coordinate the granting of allowances and support. Blackie's intent was for every member of the Guinea Pig Club to maintain their dignity despite their injuries for the rest of their lives. Edward Blacksell's loyalty to McIndoe and the Guinea Pigs was unwavering. He remained the club's Welfare Secretary all his life and held the honorary position of 'Resettlement Officer' within the Club.

12 The first newsletter published in 1994 consisted of **12** printed pages and was printed by Cullen's in Cantelupe Road, East Grinstead. The first newsletter holds no formal date but was created with a formal introduction written by Archibald McIndoe.

> 'Dear Guinea Pig.
>
> With this letter you will receive an outline of the reconstitution of the Guinea Pig Club in this copy of its first official publication. The development of this unique organisation from a meeting of the few in 1941 around a bottle of sherry to its present flourishing condition is one of the curiosities of the war. It might well have died in infancy as so many of these things have done; but instead, it has gone from strength to strength until a proper organisation has become essential. This has not been an easy task and without enthusiastic help it could never have been accomplished. I hope you approve of the result; but in case you don't your full criticism will be welcomed.
>
> I strongly believe that the same spirit that brought this club into being three years ago is still operative today and that it will grow and flower with the passage of time. It is based on the understanding that we are the trustees of each other. Most Guinea Pigs will agree that while alone they may have difficulty in holding an honoured position in the community of men, out of their united strength they can find the opportunities and facilities to achieve it. You may not yourself have "bought it" badly; but there are many who have, and it is for those less fortunate Guinea Pigs whose will to live is as strong as ever that this club really exists. We do well to remember that the privilege of dying for one's country is not equal to the privilege of living for it.
>
> With a strong and capable committee, social headquarters in London, executive headquarters in East Grinstead, a brainwave newsletter, and annual overhaul of damaged pigs, followed by dinner in East Grinstead in the true Guinea Pig style, the club will continue to make history. I hope that you will give it your support and that you will take an active part in its future development.
>
> Yours sincerely.
>
> Archibald McIndoe'[38]

2

The cover artwork on the first club newsletter boldly illustrates **2** bandaged Guinea Pigs in uniform and above them an illustration of a Spitfire adorned with D-Day invasion markings chasing a V1 Flying Bomb. The artwork was created by Henry Standen.

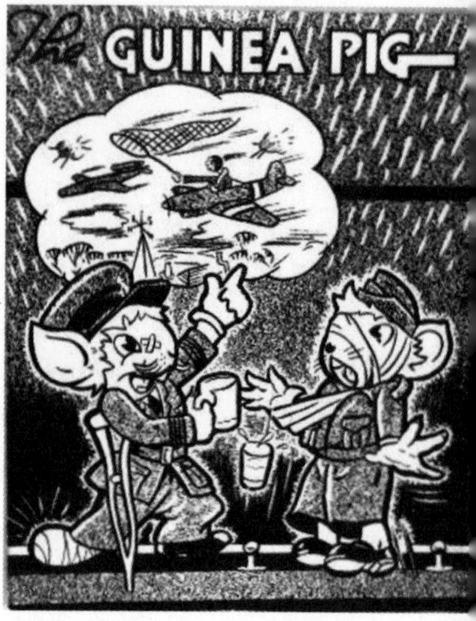

The first issue of the Guinea Pig newsletter. The illustration in the Guinea Pig's 'thought bubble' would change every issue. The Christmas 1953 issue of the magazine exposed the account of a group of Guinea Pigs who borrowed East Grinstead's fire engine. Apparently, they wanted to show it off to their fellow patients back at the Queen Victoria Hospital. Each issue often carried accounts of frivolity and humour.

12

The formal Guinea Pig Club Committee, established in 1944, consisted of **12** men. Group Captain Atcherley, Group Captain Gleave, Wing Commander Johnstone, Squadron Leader Simpson, Squadron Leader Page, Flight Lieutenant Scoffield, Flight Lieutenant Weeks, Canadian Flight Lieutenant Fredericks, Flight Lieutenant Calde, Flight Lieutenant Roberson, Warrant Officer Morris, and Flight Sergeant Standen. All were former patients in receipt of McIndoe's surgery skill over differing time periods. Flight Lieutenant Calder lost his life flying on 20 July 1944.

35

The number of individual surgical operations upon the early Hurricane pilot Guinea Pig and later 1944 committee member Peter Weeks. He went on to become the Headmaster of St Edmund's School in Hindhead, Surrey. Wing Commander Geoffrey Page was the Godfather to Week's eldest son, illustrating the strong friendship that existed between these two Guinea Pigs.

2

During recuperation after surgery Geoffrey Page and Richard Hillary both flew to the United States of America for publicity purposes. Both Guinea Pigs gave radio interviews and carried out publicity work which was of importance for war funding purposes. Richard Hillary met Edward Warburg who encouraged his writing and introduced him to the publishing world.[39] Hillary's book *The Last Enemy* was subsequently published in June 1942.

Chapter 2

The Queen Victoria Hospital

1863 This was the year that the Queen Victoria Cottage Hospital was founded, in the Sussex town of East Grinstead. At the time it was one of only **5** cottage hospitals in the country, located in Green Hedges Avenue, East Grinstead. It was little more than a converted house that only accommodated **6** beds.

1888 Twenty-four years were to elapse before the advent of the second cottage hospital which Mr and Mrs Oswald-Smith opened at their own expense on 7 January 1888. This was the year which gripped the nation with the murders associated to 'Jack the Ripper' in London.

1901 An appeal for building funds was launched in January of this year, the month in which Queen Victoria had died. In the recognition of her long reign and in her memory, the East Grinstead Cottage Hospital became the Queen Victoria Cottage Hospital.

1902 The third version of the cottage hospital was established in Queens Road, East Grinstead in this year. It was regarded as a modern facility, equipped with a Rontgen Ray, a primitive capability for what became commonly known as x ray.

1935 In this year the Army Advisory Standing Committee on Maxillo-facial Injuries, under the chairmanship of Mr J. P. Helliwell and his committee members, Mr W. Kelsey Fry, Sir Harold Gillies, and Mr Warwick James recommended the concept of a hospital solely for the special treatment of maxillo-facial injuries (severe trauma to both soft tissue and bone). This marked the dawn of dedicated surgery which would eventually be delivered at the Queen Victoria Hospital.[1]

39 Archibald McIndoe was **39** when he arrived to practice plastic surgery at the Queen Victoria Hospital. Born on 4 May 1900 in New Zealand, he had studied at the medical school of Otago University. In 1924 he was awarded a Foundation Fellowship at the Mayo Clinic, Rochester, Minnesota. He married a talented pianist on 31 July

1924 and with his wife and first daughter Adonia, named after her mother, the McIndoe family moved to Great Britain in 1931. With the assistance of Harold Gillies, he gained employment and practised at St Bartholomew's Hospital. The McIndoes second daughter, Vanora was born in London.

1936

The Peanut Club collected small charitable sums of money from the public. In this year, the club focused upon specifically helping the Queen Victoria Hospital at East Grinstead. The Peanut Club had huge success in raising thousands of pounds for the Hospital. The Peanut Club worldwide membership was estimated to be at least **350,000**.[2]

4.3

An area of land off Holtye Road was gifted to East Grinstead by the merchant banker and president of the National Savings Committee, Sir Robert Molesworth Kindersley, later Baron Kindersley of West Hoathly Sussex. The **4.3**-acre site was for a purpose-built hospital. The new Queen Victoria Cottage Hospital opened on 8 January 1936. This was effectively the fourth and final location for the hospital.

4

As war clouds darkened over Europe in the late 1930s, the Queen Victoria Hospital was selected to become one of **4** specialist Emergency Medical Service units, tasked to deal with both military and civilian casualties. The government was particularly concerned that there would be large numbers of casualties from aerial combat and air raids. In particular substantial burn injuries to both pilots and airmen was foremost in the minds of this decision making. The Ministry of Health appointed regional hospital officers, supported by county and borough medical officers of health to organise hospital services on a regional basis.

48

By March 1939, plans were in place for compliance to the desired medical service at East Grinstead. The Hospital Board of Management were tasked by the Ministry to provide for an additional capacity of patients by the accommodation of a further **48** emergency beds.

100

In May 1939, the Minister of War gave permission to erect temporary structures at the Queen Victoria Hospital in order to accommodate **100** additional beds.

33

The Queen Victoria Hospital was **33** miles from Central London. Plans were in place to evacuate all patients from the capital's hospitals as the immediate war planning progressed.

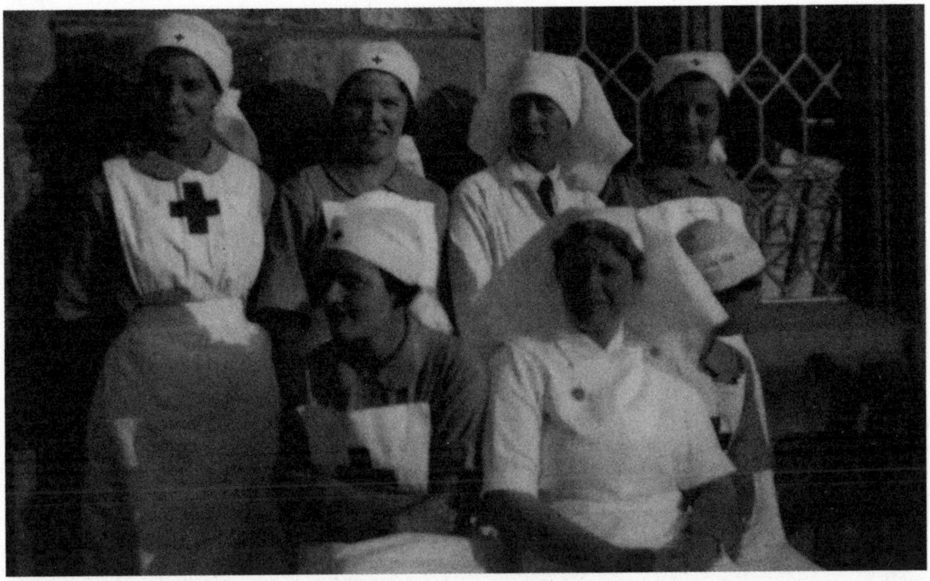

Dutton Homestall convalescence nurses.

50 The additional criteria for the hospital patients at East Grinstead was for the provision of patient convalescence capacity. Mr J. A. Dewar the whisky magnate and racehorse owner generously offered his nearby home, Dutton Homestall, as an auxiliary hospital with **50** beds in the event of war. He further undertook to finance **£4,500** per annum for the facility's requirements. Mrs Dewar was the Vice President of the British Red Cross in Sussex. Patients at the Queen Victoria Hospital also had the opportunity to convalescence at Saint Hill Manor, near East Grinstead.[3]

½ Future military patients at the Queen Victoria Hospital, and many thousands of others who signed to serve their country in recruiting centres across the country, were asked to give half of one day's pay every year for military service benevolent purposes. That benevolent fund became the provider of significant financial help to hospital structures across the country, indirectly providing assistance to every member of the Guinea Pig Club.

3 The Queen Victoria Hospital had **3** new wooden wards constructed. Ward One was intended to treat dental and jaw injuries. Ward Two was allocated for women and children, most of whom were expected to be air raid casualties or who had injuries that hospitals in London did not have capacity to deal with. Ward Three was

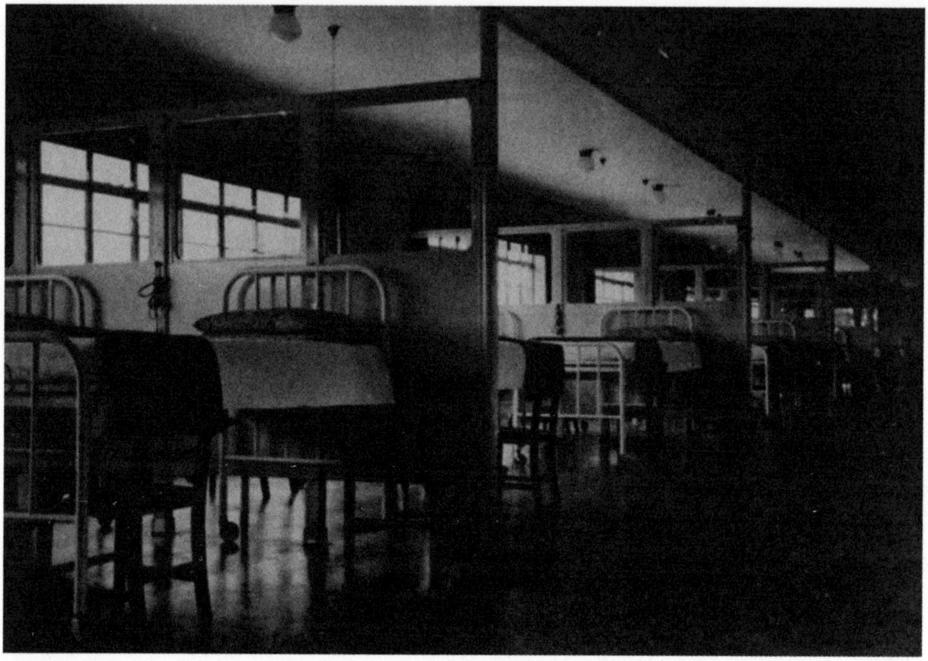

The Queen Victoria Hospital was built in 1935–6, designed by F. Gordon Troup and L. H. Parsons. The hospital had a T-shaped plan comprising a long, south-facing single ward wing and a shorter, **2**-storey support wing behind. The general wards benefitted from verandas with fully-opening windows, all facing south. The building was dominated by a tall central staircase tower. This is a view within the burn ward unit circa 1943–5. (*Australian War Memorial AWM2016.395.1.5*)

a specific medical ward set aside for officers and men amongst the most severely burned. It became a ward for providing expert treatment and surgery to men of the Royal Air Force and the other Allied and Commonwealth Air Forces.

The ward was a long low hut, with a door at one end and **20** beds facing each other along each side. It was divided into three small sections by glass partitions that rose to shoulder height. In each section were **4** beds with each bed being capable of isolation through screening and capable of being moved easily and smoothly about the wards to and from the side of the saline bath.[4]

1939

During the early hours of 1 September 1939, German troops poured over the Polish border. Great Britain, along with its allies, responded by issuing an ultimatum to Adolf Hitler, to withdraw. At 11.15 on Sunday 3 September, the voice of the Prime Minister Neville Chamberlain, speaking from Downing Street, uttered these words: 'This morning the British Ambassador in Berlin handed the German

Government a final note stating that, unless we heard from them by 11 o'clock that they were prepared at once to withdraw their troops from Poland, a state of war would exist between us. I have to tell you now, that no such undertaking has been received, and that consequently this country is at war with Germany.' Parliament immediately passed the National Service Act imposing conscription on all males aged between **18** and **41** who were required to register for military service.

4 On 4 September 1939, the day after Chamberlain's declaration of war with Germany, the Queen Victoria Hospital recorded that 'Mr McIndoe had to take over the hospital, on behalf of the Ministry of Health as a Maxillo-Facial although he had no written instructions.' McIndoe arrived at the Queen Victoria Hospital to take up his appointment as Consultant in Plastic Surgery to the RAF. He reassured the hospital board of management that he was sure the ministry would accept full financial responsibility for the financing and future running of the Hospital for the duration of the war. From 9am on 3 September 1939, Archibald McIndoe had assumed full responsibility for the hospital.[5]

3 At the outset of the Second World War, the predicted London bombings influenced McIndoe to send his wife and two children to safety in Minnesota in the United States to reside near the Mayo Clinic where he had previously practised.

4 At the outbreak of the Second World War there were just **4** fully experienced plastic surgeons in Britain: Mr Rainsford Mowlem, Professor Kilner, Sir Harold Gillies and Mr Archibald McIndoe. At the request of the government these surgeons were divided to lead **4** separate plastic surgery units to treat the expected influx of injured servicemen from the different branches of the armed services. There were another **6** plastic surgeons at the registrar level of training, these were distributed as assistants.[6] One was Alexander Burns Wallace who had met Sir Harold Gillies, Archibald McIndoe and Thomas Kilner to enhance his medical skills.[7] Wallace eventually created and edited the *British Journal of Plastic Surgery*.[8]

3 Sir Harold Gillies and Archibald McIndoe were born at Dunedin, on the South Island of New Zealand. Rainsford Mowlem was born in Auckland and studied medicine with McIndoe at the University of Otago, in Dunedin.[9] Archibald McIndoe's father, John McIndoe (1858–1916) was the son of James McIndoe and Elizabeth Gillies

(a daughter of John Gillies). Archibald McIndoe and Harold Gillies were therefore first cousins once removed.

1

William Maxwell Manchester was a junior surgeon under Gillies, and a graduate from the Otago Medical School. He was sent to the Queen Victoria Hospital on 9 December 1940.[10] William Manchester later transferred to St Albans Hospital for further training under Rainsford Mowlem and John Barron.

3

At the Queen Victoria Hospital, McIndoe was one of a specialist team of **3**. He was supported by **2** members of his regular operating theatre staff, namely his chief anaesthetist, John Hunter, and his theatre sister, Jill Mullins. As the East Grinstead Museum, website notes, 'John Hunter was considered by some as outlandish as he preferred to wear a white coat over his civilian clothes and refused to wear a surgical mask or cap for fear of looking like a "continental chef". In his work, he was imaginative as well as jolly and human in his approach. Before each operation, the good-humoured Hunter would make a bet with the [patient] that if he were sick after coming around then he would buy him a beer.' Jill Mullins had met McIndoe in 1931 while a theatre nurse at St Bartholomew's Hospital in London. Having assisted him and other surgeons including Professor Pomfret Kilner and Sir Gillies previously, she worked with tremendous efficiency and competency. In 1935, Archibald McIndoe invited her to work at his Harley Street practice. It was there that the highly skilled team of McIndoe, Hunter and Mullins came together.

210

The Queen Victoria Hospital Committee and the Sub-committee met throughout the first week of the war. With such ramifications of change imposed upon them, the board were not fully reassured by McIndoe's position or authority. Ministry directions received on 18 September 1939 declared that there was an intention to increase the beds in the main hospital to **210**.[11] The Hospital Committee were no longer influential.

30,000

A special meeting of the Hospital Board on 30 October 1939 was attended by Mr John Hunter, who was in charge of the emergency hospital scheme, Sir Harold Gillies with Mr Kelsey Fry as advisors to the Ministry of Health and Archibald McIndoe who had by that time been designated Medical Superintendent at East Grinstead. 'Mr Hunter explained that the Ministry of Health were advised that they were to expect some **30,000** casualties a week from air raids and explained at length the preparations the Ministry have made to deal with this situation.'[12] Sir Harold Gillies was influential in respect of the distribution of casualty types across the emergency hospital scheme.

1 Archibald McIndoe had been directly appointed by the Ministry of Health as the 'Medical Officer in charge of the East Grinstead Emergency Medical Scheme Section'. He held the title of Medical Superintendent.

10 On 10 May 1940, the Prime Minister Neville Chamberlain resigned. Winston Churchill formed a Coalition Government as the new Prime Minister. Sir Archibald Sinclair became the Secretary of State for Air, a post he retained until the dissolution of the coalition in May 1945.

0 In May 1940, Sir Harold Gillies was concerned that East Grinstead was receiving too many Air Force cases and recommended that casualties also be admitted to Park Prewett or Hill End Hospitals. He was keen for patients to be evacuated from East Grinstead, and to free up the hospital for the immediate treatment of air raid or invasion casualties.[13] The threat of invasion had been discussed in government since October 1939. It was not until the spring of 1940 that it was treated as a serious possibility.

46 By July 1940 the establishment of nurses at the hospital in East Grinstead was **46** and it had by then firmly established itself in delivering primarily medical services to airmen and pilots.

2 In the early hours of 3 June 1940, the people in and around the Queen Victoria Hospital were woken by **2** shattering explosions. Two aerial mines had been dropped near Heasman's Mead in Forest Row. This incident commenced a period of bombing by both day and night in and around the district of East Grinstead, including the immediate geographical areas of Imberhorn, Crawley Down, Copthorne, Turners Hill, Forest Row and West Hoathly.

14 On 13 September 1940, one Luftwaffe bomber dropped a string of **14** bombs from the railway station at nearby Forest Row, into Hartfield Road and Station Road. Properties were damaged and **2** people were killed.[14] The daylight raids by the German air force that day also targeted Buckingham Palace. The King and Queen escaped injury whist **3** palace staff were injured.

1

A Luftwaffe bomber on 26 September 1940, crashed onto the residence of Angus Simpson of North End, East Grinstead. It had been taking part in a bombing mission to London. One of the German airman, A. Brautigam had parachuted out injured and was admitted to the Queen Victoria Hospital. A second crewman H. Winkelmann had also parachuted out and was admitted to the hospital but he died on the following day. The failure of crew member R. Precht's parachute caused his death and he fell in the area of Hartfield, approximately **8** miles distant of East Grinstead. The Luftwaffe pilot, H. Kasing, died in the aircraft. The Simpsons' house was cut in half but miraculously nobody was injured from that household.[15] The Ju 88 bomber from the unit 3/KG77 3Z+BL had been shot down by Squadron Leader E. A. McNab, American Flying Officer De Peyster Douw Brown, Pilot Officer B. E. Christmas and the Polish Pilot Officer J. E. L. Zumbach at 9.20pm.

1

The first nurse working at the Queen Victoria Hospital that lost her life to enemy bombing occurred on Saturday 26 October 1940. Forty-nine-year-old Nurse Dorothy Parsons was resident at a property called 'Stanney' in Holtye Road. At 9pm she was in the bath when the property was destroyed by a bomb. **3** other lady occupants were trapped in the rubble but uninjured, whilst the bathing nurse was also buried but terribly injured. The rescue party extracted the nurse who was taken to the Larches nursing home where Doctor Somerville and his staff did what was possible. The nurse however died the following day in the Queen Victoria Hospital. Dorothy was a State Registered Nurse.[16]

20

Towards the end of 1940, Archibald McIndoe commenced the training of surgeons at the Queen Victoria Hospital. He addressed the fundamentals of plastic surgery and jaw injuries combined with burn cases. On average, an estimated **20** surgeons a year were thereafter to pass through the hospital. Nursing sisters also underwent short attachments at East Grinstead as did nursing orderlies.

1

To identify staff employed at the Queen Victoria Hospital under the emergency measures, a blue and white enamel badge was worn. This identified them as part of the Emergency Hospitals Service. They were part of Britain's wartime Civil Defence structure, staffed mainly by the Civil Nursing Reserve and employed by the Ministry of Health.

1 A Luftwaffe Dornier bomber was shot down and crashed at Lower Sheriffs Cottages, West Hoathley, approximately **5** miles from East Grinstead. **2** crewmen were killed, **1** was captured and the final airman, E. Nurnberg, who had been badly wounded in the aircraft crash, was admitted to East Grinstead Hospital.

235 Winifred Dorothy Catterick appears to have been the second nurse who lost her life to the enemy bombing. Winifred was 39 and resided at Pixiewood, in Stream Park, Felbridge. Working as a registered nurse at the Hospital, Winifred was killed in the tragic Whitehall Cinema bombing around 5pm on 9 July 1943. Winifred was buried on 14 July 1943 in one of the two communal graves at Mount Noddy, the main cemetery for East Grinstead for victims of the Whitehall bombing. **235** people were injured in the bombing and **108** were killed. It was the largest loss of life in any air raid in Sussex during the Second World War. The town of East Grinstead saw a load of some **12** bombs dropped, **2** of which failed to explode.

7 The Queen Victoria Hospital featured significantly in treating the Whitehall casualties, **7** of whom died in the hospital during the following weeks. Doreen Joan Barrett was injured at the Whitehall Cinema on 9 July 1943 and died at the Queen Victoria Hospital the same day. Kate Walden Tooth, lived at Forest View High Street, East Grinstead, injured at Forest View, 9 July and died at Queen Victoria Hospital, the same day. Francis Gordon Currie of 7, Beeches Fields, Ashurst Wood, was injured in the bombing on 9 July and died at Queen Victoria Hospital the following day. Edwin Tooth husband of Kate Walden Tooth, injured at Forest View, 9 July, died at Queen Victoria Hospital, on 10 July 1943. Erica Fothergill lived at 'The Beacon' Dormansland, was injured in London Road on 9 July, and died at Queen Victoria Hospital, 12 July 1943. Frederick Albert Brooker lived at 4 West View Gardens, East Grinstead. He was a Leading Fireman in the National Fire Service. Injured in the High Street on 9 July, he died at Queen Victoria Hospital on 18 July 1943. Ethel Smith who lived at 66 Dorset Avenue, East Grinstead, was injured in the cinema bombing and lost her life **5** days after her admission to the hospital aged 30.[17]

The Queen Victoria Hospital was responsible for caring for the deceased bodies until they could be properly identified. Multiple casualties with crush and burn injuries were treated. Percy Jayes the resident medical officer to Archibald McIndoe at the Queen Victoria Hospital acted as the lead with the hospital staff working

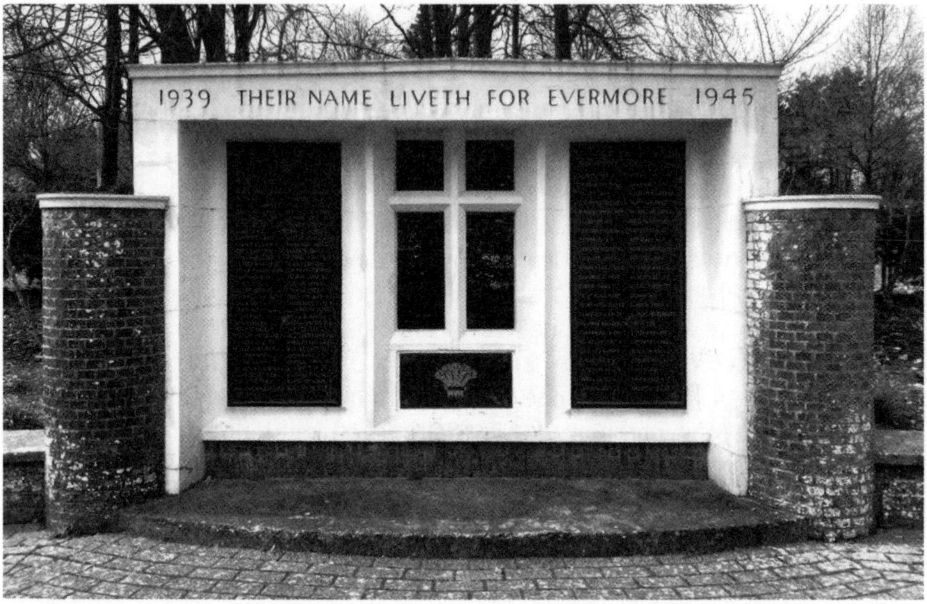

The East Court Estate in East Grinstead was bought by a local merchant banker and philanthropist, Alfred Wagg, through a Charitable Trust in September 1945. The intent was to provide grounds and a memorial to the men, women and children of East Grinstead who lost their lives in the 1939–45 war, the significant loss of life at the Whitehall Cinema building no doubt being instrumental to the cause. Alfred Wagg engaged with and supported the Queen Victoria Hospital. The memorial sits within the grounds and seating provides long reaching views towards Ashdown Forrest.

throughout the day and night in all available operating theatres.[18] It was not possible to positively identify all those who died at the scene of the bombing. A report of the East Grinstead raid state that 'In spite of the heavy loss of life incurred by the bombing of the local cinema the morale of the people is described as sound. The tragedy is accepted, albeit sorrowfully, as an unlucky chance. The Civil Defence workers and the local troops who helped to clear the debris are praised, and there is said to have been no criticism of the defences or anyone else. The most painful scenes were at the improvised mortuary where the difficult task of identification was proceeding.'[19]

2

Nurse Frances Mary Long a Voluntary Aid Detachment (VAD) nurse at the Queen Victoria Hospital, was also killed in the Whitehall cinema bombing on 9 July 1943. Mary and her mother both lost their lives sitting together in the auditorium. They were buried together at the Mount Noddy cemetery in Blackwell Road, East Grinstead.

6 The number of Royal Canadian Air Force Nurses serving at the Queen Victoria Hospital prior to the Canadian Wing construction.

1 Sir Harold Gillies was practising at Park Prewett Hospital near Basingstoke. The plastic surgery unit was within Park Prewett's Rooksdown House. Gillies in his role as Consultant Advisor to the Ministry of Health, travelled around the country inspecting hospitals and writing reports.[20]

1 Susie Bergeau was a cook at the Whitehall restaurant as well as a volunteer at the Queen Victoria Hospital blood transfusion group. Regional blood depots were established throughout the country. The depots, which later became known as the Regional Transfusion Centres were managed by the Emergency Medical Service.

25 The number of Royal Canadian Air Force nurses known to have served primarily in the Canadian Wing at the Queen Victoria Hospital. They were: Frances Oakes, Marjorie Jackson, Leonora Mardell, Elaine Matheson, Enid Faulkner, Hilda Emke, Maggie Kaines, Frances Anderson, Olwen Gregory, Bee Phillips, Ina Bishop, Helen Brown, Bernie Arnell, Dorothy Mulholland, Marion Patterson, Margaret Peacock, Eileen Angley, Midge Phillps, Sara McLellan, Marjorie Stapleford, Mabel Gardner, Lilian Hand, Shirley Williams, Mary Philllps and Lillian Hall.

1 Mollie Lentaigne, the renown Medical Artist was a VAD nurse at the Queen Victoria Hospital between 1941 and 1945.

1 Monique Agazarian became a nurse with the VAD stationed at the Royal Air Force station at Uxbridge. She also nursed at the Queen

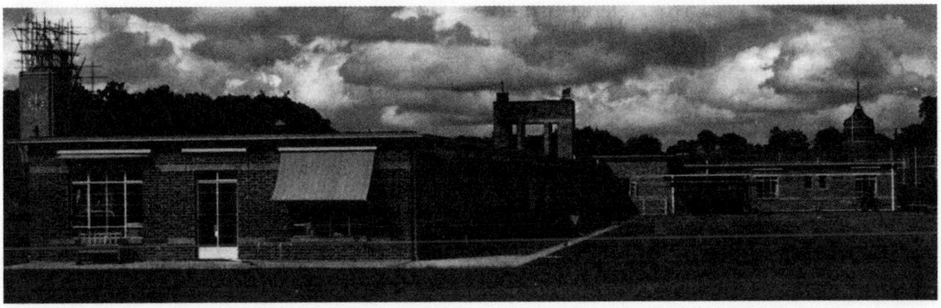

The Canadian Wing built at the Queen Victoria Hospital in 1944. Canadian patients occupied the new wing in July that year. Thereafter orders stated that any Canadian who needed plastic surgery should be brought to the East Grinstead Hospital. (*Canadian Weekly* 14.9.45.)

Victoria Hospital before later being accepted for training to become a pilot for the Air Transport Auxiliary in 1943. As a pilot she flew many assorted aircraft between airfields across Great Britain.

2

Rosemary Kerr and Beryl Daintry were both Ward Three VAD nurses at the Queen Victoria Hospital.

8

The number of Ward Three nurses known by forenames only. They were Gladys, Alice, Mary, Joyce, Irene, Violet, Anita and Bridget.[21]

1

Matron Caroline Hall was in charge of the nursing staff at the hospital throughout the war years.

1

East Grinstead remained an Emergency Medical Scheme hospital throughout the war. The hospital had **1** of the highest levels of nursing staff. A large proportion of those nurses were Red Cross Nurses and VAD nurses. Whilst not as experienced as professional civilian or military nurses, VAD nurses were vital in sharing the demanding workload.[22]

2

Archibald McIndoe wrote **2** research articles at the Queen Victoria Hospital in 1943. They were '*Rehabilitation in a Maxillo Facial and Plastic Centre*' and '*Skin Grafting in the Treatment of Wounds*'.[23]

2

Celia Liggins and Pamela Martin were both Red Cross nurses who served in Ward Three. Pamela frequently nursed Frankie Truhlar and voluntarily spent time supporting him out in the community.[24]

1

There was a Royal Air Force Registrar serving at the East Grinstead Hospital, namely Squadron Leader G. Morley. It is assumed he was working with Percy Jayes the resident medical officer to Archibald McIndoe at the hospital.

12

On 12 August 1940, the board of the Queen Victoria Hospital unanimously agreed to the resolution that 'the Board would not in future accept any financial responsibility resulting from action taken by the Medical Superintendent [Archibald McIndoe]'.[25]

2,000

Winston Churchill announced in the House of Commons that during the first half of September 1940 about **2,000** civilians had been killed and **8,000** had been injured in the air bombardment by the Luftwaffe. The Luftwaffe bombing blitz had seen Archibald Ball, a soldier admitted to the Queen Victoria Hospital on 28 October

1940. Suffering facial and foot injuries he had been taken directly to East Grinstead hospital. He received **3** operations to his injuries and despite serving as an Army Soldier, he is recorded as a verified member of the Guinea Pig Club.[26]

12 Saint Hill Manor a significant building near East Grinstead, occupied by Mr and Mrs Neville Laskey opened its doors providing **12** beds for convalescing RAF patients.[27]

4 Elaine Laskey of Saint Hill Manor became a widower and later married Neville Blond of Gotwick Manor, Hammerwood, a residence some **4** miles east of East Grinstead. Her first husband had been a cousin of Neville Blond, a textile manufacturer and philanthropist. A friendship with Archibald McIndoe resulted in the Blonds opening their Sussex home to convalescing Guinea Pig patients. Elaine was one of the main organisers of the pre-war Kindertransport's extraction of children from Germany. After the war she played a prominent role on the 'Committee for the Care of the Concentration Camp Children'.[28] She was the third daughter of Michael Marks, the Russian-Polish immigrant who founded Marks and Spencer.

2 By the end of 1940, the Dental Department at the Queen Victoria Hospital occupied a spacious wooden building. A second hut for the accommodation of the resident medical officer was erected, that building bears the name of Percy Lodge, a dedication to its occupant, Percy Jayes, who later became a consultant plastic surgeon to the hospital.

1 Dorothy Crighton, known as 'Teddy', was a voluntary driver at the Queen Victoria Hospital. She named her vehicles 'Brown Cow' and 'Grey Mare'. These were the vehicles which often transported nurses to and from numerous hostels and other accommodation facilities. It has to be assumed that they also transported Guinea Pigs to the various recouperation locations around the proximity of the hospital.

1 There was **1** wartime Red Cross Recreational Hut within the grounds of the Queen Victoria Hospital. It was open all hours, staffed by volunteers George Godfrey, Jack Bright, Mrs Spalding and Mrs Beal. During the summer of 1941, the orderlies would push bedridden patients out onto the lawn alongside the ward. They would be able to look up and watch the squadrons of Spitfires as they passed overhead to carry out fighter sweeps over France.

4 The number of dental surgeons on site at the hospital in 1940. They were W. Kelsey Fry, D. G. Walker, A. C. McLeod and A. H. Clarkson.

1 During 1941, Sister Mary Rae was the night nurse in Ward Three at the Queen Victoria Hospital. She also served as night nurse at Dutton Homestall before becoming a regular member of the operating staff in the hospital's surgical theatres. Mary was very popular amongst the Guinea Pigs. She proudly wore her Friend of the Guinea Pig Club Badge in the post-war years.

1 Archibald McIndoe initially resided at the property Little Warren in Luxford Lane on the outskirts of East Grinstead.

1 A convalescent annex opened in July 1941 at the School House of St. Agnes' Convent, East Grinstead. This had been made possible through the co-operation of the Mother Superior when the Queen Victoria Hospital received more cases than the original scheme was designed to cope with. The Ministry of Health agreed to this development.[29]

4,500 Between 1939 and 1945 there were over **4,500** Allied airmen who suffered burn injuries.[30] Severe burns would often initiate a chain reaction of events beginning with fluid loss from the wound, followed by shock and the successive failure of multiple organ systems until the patient was no longer able to cling to life. Archibald McIndoe used baths filled with saline and plasma, a technique first developed in the 1930s, which kept aviators from becoming dehydrated. Daily saline baths helped to keep healing skin flexible and adaptable for the skin grafts that McIndoe and his staff deployed to repair the damaged skin tissue. McIndoe was skilled in harvesting sheets of tissue paper-thin skin grafts, using an open razor with a 10in blade. An item which had to be stropped for sharpness and re-sterilised for each use.[31]

2 The Royal Air Force Medical Services circulated **2** memoranda from Archibald McIndoe forbidding the use of tannic acid derivatives upon burn injuries in October 1940. This instruction was reiterated in February 1941.[32]

0 There were no qualified psychiatrists on the medical staff at the Queen Victoria Hospital. Archibald McIndoe treated the minds of his patients unorthodoxly but with apparent unrivalled success. The

Royal Air Force Hospital Matlock, located in Derbyshire was the requisitioned building which was used as a psychiatric facility for 'disturbed' airmen. It was treating and rehabilitating aircrew and ground personnel in a closed environment.[33]

60 David Matthews, a consultant plastic surgeon at the Westminster Hospital, became Archibald McIndoe's first assistant at the plastic surgery unit at the Queen Victoria Hospital. In 1939 Matthews spent three days a week in Sussex and four at the London Westminster. He later accepted a commission in the Royal Air Force Volunteer Reserve and in 1941 he took charge of the **60**-bed plastic surgery unit at Royal Air Force Halton. It was at Halton where Matthews wrote *The Surgery of Repair Injuries and Burns* in 1943.

4 In 1941 **4** hospitals Halton in Buckinghamshire, Ely in Cambridgeshire, Rauceby in Lincolnshire and Cosford in Staffordshire became burn injury centres. Each was led by surgeons who had undergone courses with McIndoe at East Grinstead. Each hospital had around **12** beds and **2** saline baths. Patient's injuries were photographed as treatments progressed. The images were ideal for medical staff consultation. Each centre was equipped with Leica cameras, a clinical photographer, dark room and enlarging apparatus. Standardised views of different parts of the body were taken to

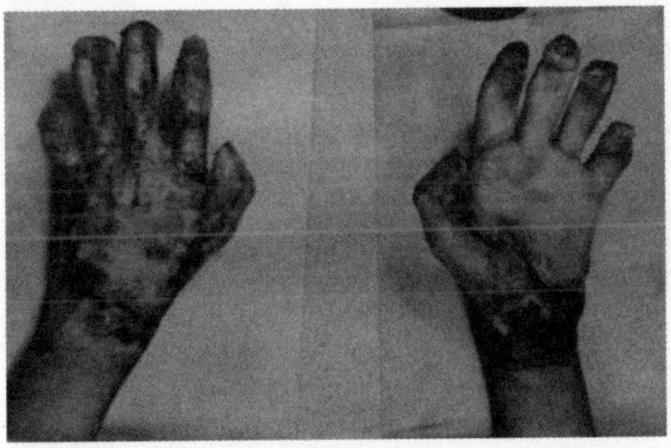

Above: Burn injuries to the hands of Sid McQuillan.

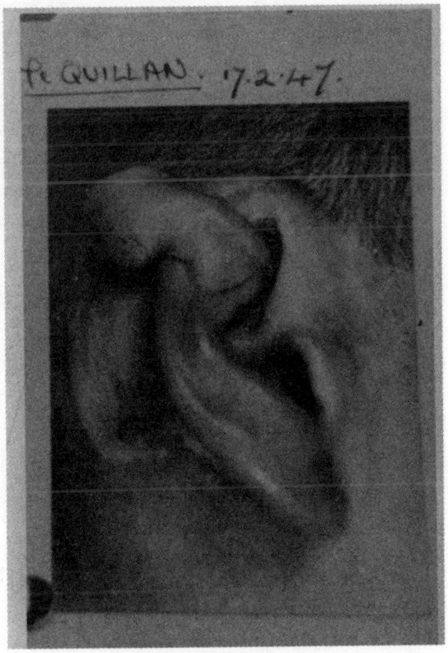

Right: The ear pedicle skin graft creating new skin for Sid McQuillan's post-war treatments at the Queen Victoria Hospital. The surgeon created a pedicle tube by making **2** parallel incisions and then stitching the edges into a tube. Surgeons could move the new tissue growth in gradual steps from the donor site to the wound.

display the extent and as far as possible, the depth of burns. Hands, for example, were photographed to display and record the extent of the range of function of the fingers. The clinical photographer also copied and reduced X-ray films for inclusion in the records of the orthopaedic department.[34]

1

Fenton Braithwaite at Rauceby welcomed Archibald McIndoe who visited at least twice a month. Together they worked in the crash and burns unit which was located in Orchard House at Rauceby. Braithwaite had accepted a commission in the RAF for the duration of the war, becoming the officer in charge of the Surgical Division at Rauceby, Lincolnshire with the rank of Wing Commander. Rauceby's clinical photographer was Bill Howlett. The theatre sister who worked alongside Braithwaite and McIndoe was Nan Hunter. Fenton Braithwaite was later awarded the Military Division of the Order of the British Empire for his work.

3

This was the number of daily saline baths that were often deployed to any single patient at the Queen Victoria Hospital. This bathing kept the healing skin flexible which made it receptive to skin grafts.

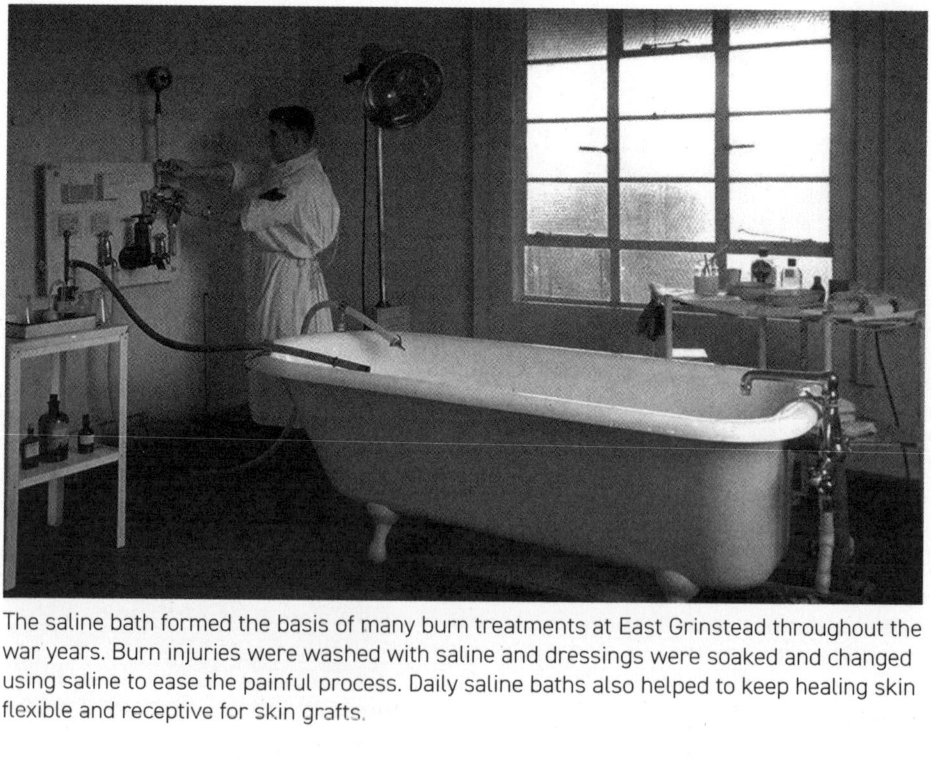

The saline bath formed the basis of many burn treatments at East Grinstead throughout the war years. Burn injuries were washed with saline and dressings were soaked and changed using saline to ease the painful process. Daily saline baths also helped to keep healing skin flexible and receptive for skin grafts.

6 The number of East Grinstead Ward Three saline bath staff. They were Flight Sergeant Salmon, and Corporals Bernie Hollins, Johnnie Dawkins, Frank Teague, Eddie Downey and Betty Andrews. Each bath was required to be effectively isolated or earthed as any metal parts were subjected to electrical conductivity caused by the saline. Each bath facility required stretchers or ward beds to access and facilitate patients being lifted without obstruction. After the patient was lifted out of the bath the burn areas were cleansed, dusted with sulphonamide powder and covered with tulle gras dressings before skin grafting could be undertaken. This work required heavy lifting and the male nursing orderlies were required for undertaking those tasks including the maintenance and general nursing services of the saline bath units which was intensive.

1 Cyril Ashton was in charge of the saline bath in Ward Four at East Grinstead.

7 The number of types of skin grafts deployed by the surgeons at the Queen Victoria Hospital: Pedicle graft, Stamp graft, Pinch graft, Flap graft, Dermatome graft, Thiersch graft and the Wolfe graft.[35]

1 Archibald McIndoe possessed a love of music and was a fine pianist. A piano in Ward Three, which may well have been purloined by McIndoe, was often played by him.

3 The Queen Victoria Hospital introduced physical separation of the **3** units holding burn casualties from all other wards of the hospital. This served to reduce infection rates created by cross-contamination among different patient groups. Patients with the highest risk of infection were those with burn wounds and jaw injuries.

1 In January 1941 a serious outbreak of streptococcal infection spread through Ward Three. Many grafts failed and infection spread, leading to the movement of patients into Dewar ward. This unfortunate outbreak resulted in the progression towards a dedicated pathological department being created at the hospital.[36]

115 Between the start of the war and up to January 1941, this number of jaw fractures had been operated upon successfully.[37]

8 Many injured airmen could be in the hospital for lengthy periods. It was customary to plan **8** surgeries per patient per year, alternating

3 to **4** weeks in hospital, with **2**-to-**3**-week recuperation breaks before readmittance.

1

A large single Luftwaffe bomb fell in the grounds of the hospital on 17 February 1941 which failed to explode. Sandbag protection to the wards was put in place and some patents were removed to Dutton Homestall. Geoffrey Page in his book *Tale of a Guinea Pig* states he recognised from the beat of the engines that the aircraft dropping the bomb was a Junkers Ju 88. The bomb struck the ground, shaking the hospital building. Had the bomb exploded it would have created significant casualties as the blast would have been unhindered and relatively close to the wards. The local newspaper stated that the bomb affected evacuation in Holtye Road and the hospital locality. Once disabled the bomb was displayed in the town for several weeks in aid of a war charity.[38]

0

There was no RAF rank structure or seniority in Ward Three. Officers and non-commissioned airmen mixed without restriction. It was a unique and transformative environment, like no other which any patient had ever experienced, primarily because when operational, commissioned officers were separated from non-commissioned personnel in every sense and in all environments. Only in the air, flying as a crew was a non-commissioned pilot in charge regardless of officer status.

4

In 1943, **4** prestigious visitors visited the Queen Victoria Hospital. The visits of Clement Attlee the deputy prime minister, Harold Balfour of the Air Ministry, William Astor and Harold Nicolson were reported upon in the *East Grinstead Gazette*. In 1940, Harold Nicolson had been appointed a Junior Minister under Winston Churchill. He apparently acted as an unofficial link between the government and the Free French until the war ended.

40

The patient trolley which carried Guinea Pigs into theatre was manoeuvred for many years by theatre orderly Cyril Jones. Cyril became a confidant to the patients and he frequently socialised with them. His name is referenced in the Guinea Pig Club newsletters and always in complimentary terms. Cyril Jones served at the Queen Victoria Hospital for **40** years.

10

In early 1941, Archibald McIndoe was performing on average **10** operations each day.[39]

2 The number of floors of the Middlesex Hospital in London that housed the Royal Air Force Central Medical Establishment. This was where the medical board assessments were undertaken to establish if the patient could be posted operational after hospitalisation. Guinea Pigs were often faced with limited ability and inevitably if fit, posted to ground duties. Being invalided out of service completely was avoided if possible. Inevitably injured air crew often requested flying duties. Accepting that combat flying was unlikely to be authorised, they willingly undertook any form of service flying.

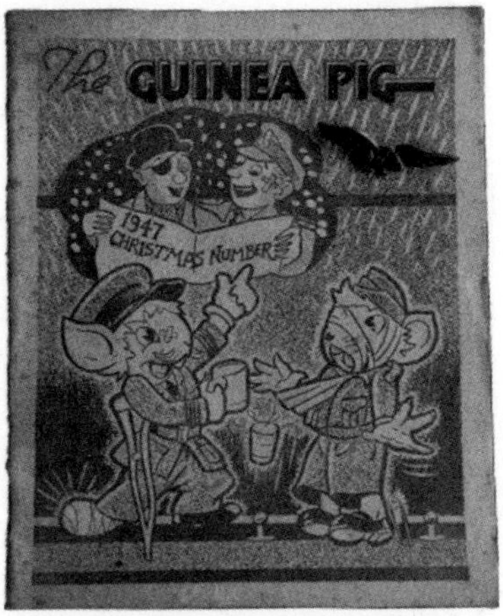

The Guinea Pig newsletter and membership badge. The cover illustrating the inset bubble content by the character's unpreaching arm.

1 Any person invalided out of service would have been able to wear 'The King's Badge' which was worn only on civilian clothing. It was issued by the British government to persons who had been discharged through injury due to war service, sometimes referred to as a wound badge. This small silver circular badge had the crowned monogram of the King in the centre, and around the edge it stated 'For Loyal Service'. It was a rather insignificant badge and it was something which Archibald McIndoe took upon himself to avoid being issued to his Guinea Pigs.

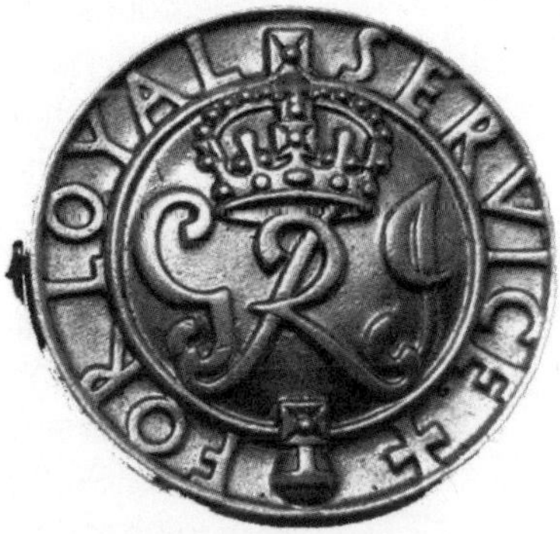

The King's Badge issued by the pensions department to every member of military who was removed from service through injuries.

13 In January 1942, the club held its first informal reunion dinner at the Whitehall, East Grinstead. The reunion dinner event continued to be held at the Whitehall for the following **13** years.

1942

In March of this year, directions were issued by the Canadian Ministry of Health to all Emergency Medical Service hospitals and medical installations for all Canadian personnel requiring plastic or maxillo-facial treatment to be transferred to East Grinstead Hospital.[40]

1

The Duke of Kent, wearing his RAF Air Commodore's uniform as the senior Welfare Officer to the service, visited the Queen Victoria Hospital on several occasions. On 25 August 1942, His Royal Highness Prince George, Duke of Kent, and his entourage lost their lives when their aircraft crashed into a hillside on a remote headland near Dunbeath in Caithness, Scotland, while flying to Iceland.

1942

Group Captain Albert Ross Tilley the Canadian medical surgeon arrived at East Grinstead in this year. Tilley was one of the first Canadian physicians to train in plastic surgery. He had become the principal Canadian Air Force medical officer in 1941. Tilley commenced working alongside Archibald McIndoe, perfecting and developing surgical techniques by shadowing the latter. Tilley became an integral part of the burns and plastic surgery unit and in due course was instrumental in creating a dedicated Canadian contingent of the Guinea Pig Club. Doctor Ross Tilley was a fervent advocate for all of the airmen in his care. They affectionately referred to him as 'Wingco'. Archibald McIndoe was likewise addressed by his patients as 'The Maestro'.

7

The total number of Canadian personnel at the hospital in July 1942, when the first all-Canadian medical team operation was formed .[41] A further nursing sister was added to the Canadian establishment in October 1942 and in the spring of 1943, **2** nursing orderlies, who were to be trained in the special technique of saline baths and care of burns, arrived at East Grinstead.

38

During 1942, **38** Canadian aircrew cases and **16** readmissions were admitted to East Grinstead Hospital.

20

Spitfire pilot Robert Fraser was more than likely the first Canadian pilot to lose his right arm in an amputation following a flying accident. Suffering severe facial injuries he arrived at the East Grinstead hospital on 23 July 1942. Another aircraft had landed across his path causing a catastrophic collision. The injuries sustained required some **20** operations in reconstructive surgery, including bone grafting to his nose.[42]

50 Such was the number of Canadian patients at East Grinstead, that Wing Commander Tilley influenced the Canadian government to fund the building of a dedicated Canadian Wing at the hospital. Tilley desired a building with a capacity for **50** beds for the treatment of Canadian airmen.

1 At mid-day on 26 October 1942, East Grinstead saw **1** Luftwaffe bomber drop a string of bombs across the West Hill and Brooklands estate. Considerable damage was done to several locations but by great good fortune nobody was killed. Another enemy bomber crossed the Channel at the same time and was reported to have dropped **4** bombs near Rochford Hospital.

£20,000 In June 1943, the Canadian Government granted this sum of money towards the cost of the Canadian building which was to be erected on land bought by the Peanut Club. On 11 December 1943, the foundation stone was laid by Air Marshal Sir Harold Edwards in the presence of Mr Atlee, Deputy Prime Minister, and other officials.[43]

50 The assistance of the Royal Canadian Engineers was enlisted for construction, and the work was begun in September 1943. The **50**-bed Canadian Wing opened in 1944. Marjorie Jackson became the

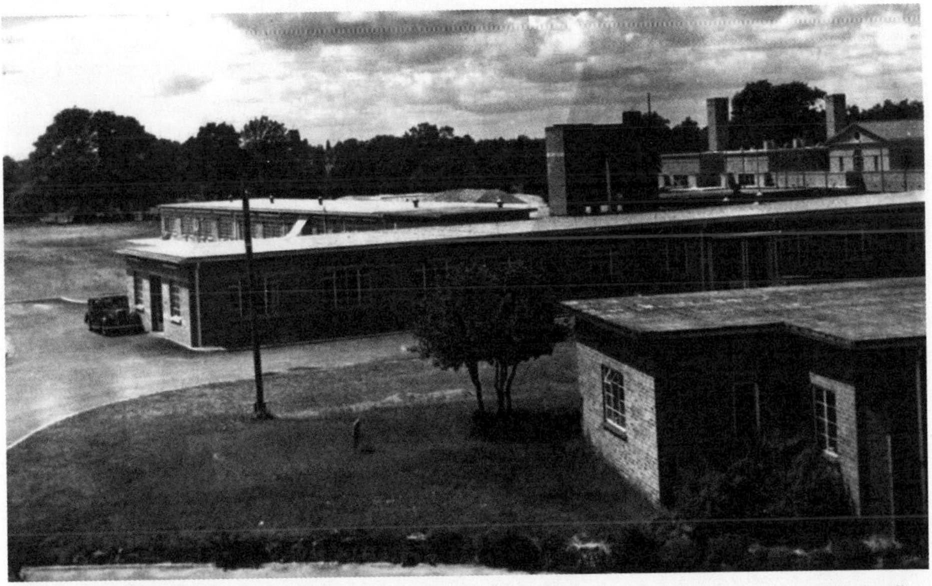

The Canadian Wing. The Canadian government supplied the funding, while the Royal Canadian Engineers built the wing. When it opened in the summer of 1944, the wing had **50** beds, **2** saline baths, and a staff of **51** medical personnel. (*Canadian Weekly* 14.9.45.)

Matron in the Canadian Wing. Building maintenance thereafter was the responsibility of the Queen Victoria Hospital.

1 The Canadian Wing Medical Liaison Officer Doctor Norman Park had arrived at East Grinstead in 1942. He subsequently served as an anaesthetist alongside Doctor J Arthur Peart until the end of the war. The Canadian Doctors George Bateman and John Hilz were also resident in the Canadian Wing.

£50,000 Lloyds of London the leading marketplace for insurance gifted this sum of money to the Royal Air Force Benevolent Fund in 1943. A direction required that the money should be spent upon welfare needs within **20** years of being gifted. The Queen Victoria Hospital Guinea Pig Club was a specified recipient within this funding.[44]

1 The known number of Merchant Navy sailors admitted to the Queen Victoria Hospital. Alexander Donald Allen became a patient having suffered burns on board an unidentified ship and received treatment

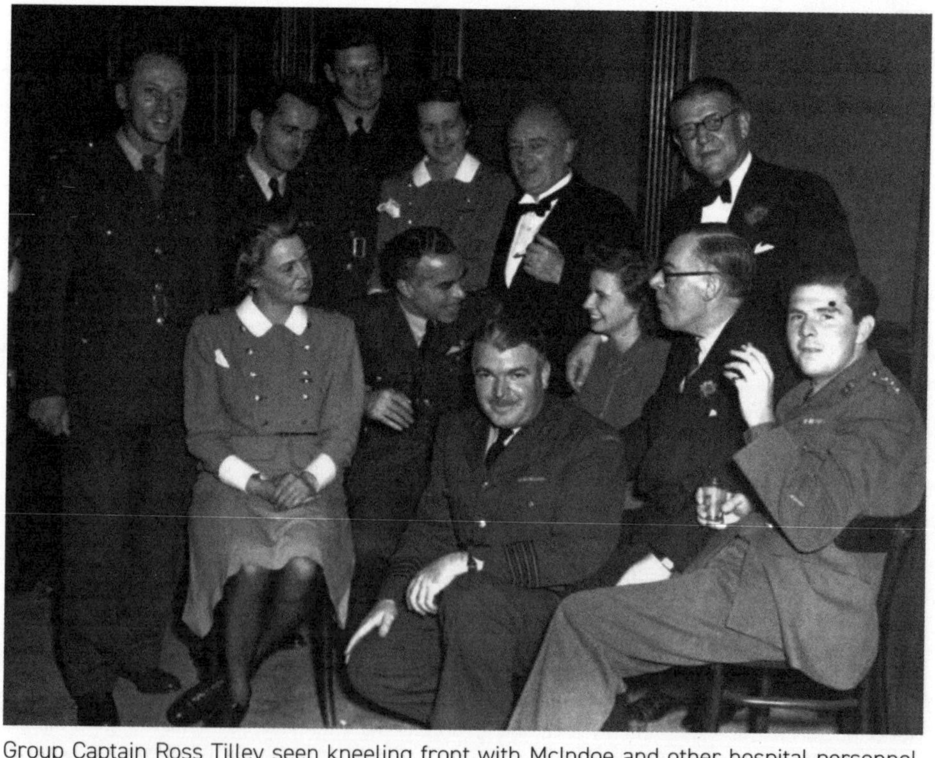

Group Captain Ross Tilley seen kneeling front with McIndoe and other hospital personnel. Thought to have been taken in 1945.

by Archibald McIndoe in 1944. He was not recorded as becoming a Guinea Pig. He did, however, become an official friend of the club which he heartily supported throughout the post-war years.

51 The newly-completed Canadian wing saw an increasing number of Canadian medical personnel employed, increasing from **7** to **51**. There were **18** officers consisting of the commanding officer, senior surgeon, an assistant surgeon, an anaesthetist, **1** other medical officer, a matron and **12** nursing sisters, all of whom were commissioned officers. In addition, there was a women's division messing officer and **33** other ranks, of whom **15** were women serving as medical clerks, hospital chefs, hospital and laboratory assistants and general duty personnel. Ross Tilley in charge of the Canadian Wing was promoted to the rank of Group Captain.

1 In 1944 Ross Tilley was appointed an Officer of the Order of the British Empire, and by appointment he was presented to King George VI at Buckingham Palace when the award was bestowed on him that summer.

2,300 Archibald McIndoe recorded in his minute book that he had performed no less than this number of operations over 1941 to 1942 and he was becoming troubled by some hand discomfort.[45]

2 Doctors George Bateman and John Hiltz both assisted Ross Tilley in the Canadian Wing operating theatres.

6 Sydney Noyes, burnt during flying training on 24 May 1942, was amongst a group of **6** Canadian Guinea Pigs, who whilst recuperating between medical operations, engaged in civil engineering work. They assisted in the building of air sea rescue launches at the Carrier Engineering works in Wembley London. Archibald McIndoe regarded the 'loaning out' of his patients as beneficial to any facilities that welcomed the Guinea Pigs.

25 Archibald McIndoe created **25** work stations for rehabilitation work in what was known as the 'Industrial Therapy Unit' at the Queen Victoria Hospital. Patients were employed to construct delicate aircraft instruments in works contracted to the hospital by George Reid for the Ministry of Aircraft Production.

60 East Grinstead was delegated as the training environment for all service dental surgeons throughout the war. In respect of plastic surgery, Archibald McIndoe had trained **60** surgeons by the middle of 1943.

1 Surgeon Nigel Dutt was an RAF Medical Officer who became a surgeon after training at East Grinstead under Archibald McIndoe. Nigel Dutt married a theatre nurse only identified by her first name, Dorothy. He served in the post-war years becoming a recognised expert in his chosen field of medical expertise.[46]

1943 In September 1943, it was officially decided to remove the word 'Cottage' from the hospital title with the approval of the Board of Trade.

1 A medical condition called 'Dupuytrens Contractures' affected Archibald McIndoe's left hand in 1943. Fellow surgeon Rainsford Mowlem was consulted and he undertook the delicate operation on McIndoe's digital nerves. Mowlem released the contractures for Archibald successfully.[47]

3 Sir Harold Gillies, Rainsford Mowlen, and Archibald McIndoe were the **3** partners in private practice at 149 Harley Street, London. Their contact at Harley Street was by telegram and cables to 'Plastisurg' London. Rainsford Mowlen operated at Hill End Hospital, St Albans during the war and he had the distinction of engaging with penicillin trials at that location.[48]

1943 In this year, Archibald McIndoe was admitted to a London hospital for abdominal surgery. Wing Commander Tilley assumed command of the Queen Victoria Hospital. McIndoe's fear of cancer was alleviated as his operation resulted in the removal of his appendix. His recovery was, however, problematic, caused by a theatre assistant inadvertently leaving a swab sponge in his abdomen.[49]

4 The Queen Victoria hospital's Sister in Ward Four between 1944 and 1946 was Marjorie Ramsden.[50]

2 The hospital's Ward One Sister was Mary Davis. The Canadian Wing Staff nurse during the war years was Kathleen McIvor.

7 The patient who occupied Bed **7** in Ward Three during the war years presumably received gift parcels sent from South Africa by Mrs L.

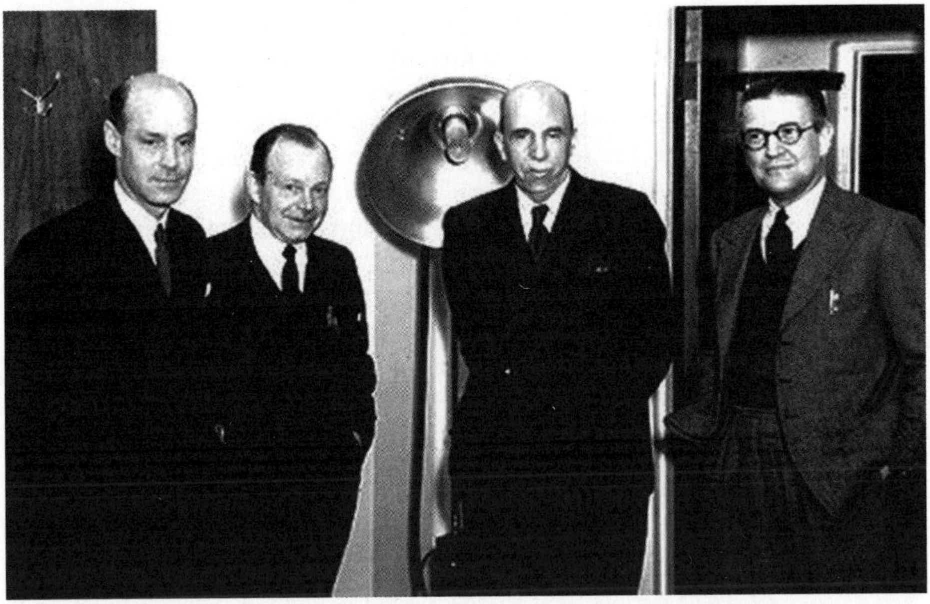

Surgeons Rainsford Mowlem, Thomas Kilner, Harold Gillies and Archibald McIndoe. The location and date are unknown. (*Image provided by BAPRAS Martin Coady*)

M. Robertson of Hermanus, south-east of Cape Town, South Africa. This friend of the Guinea Pigs was responsible for innumerable assorted parcels which were distributed to everyone. The connection to Bed Seven remains unknown.[51] The Queen Victoria Hospital admitted ten South African Air Force patients into its wards. None of those particular Guinea Pigs appear to have any connection to Mrs Robertson.

0

Occurrences exist where records relating to Guinea Pigs are lost, missing or contain errors. This explains why the register or listings of entitled club membership numbers carry differences. Some forenames in particular those of Polish members differ. The Polish Leading Aircraftsman, Czeslaw Prusski is also referenced as Creslay. He was a Guinea Pig who received surgery to his foot at the Queen Victoria Hospital.[52]

61

The number of Guinea Pigs who endured **10** or more operations at East Grinstead.

5

The number of Guinea Pigs who were operated upon between **40** to **60** occasions.

97

The number of Guinea Pigs who are recorded as having undergone one medical operation at East Grinstead.[53]

80

The highest record of operations performed on any patient at East Grinstead. Australian Charles Gamble Doria Butler, a soldier with the Australian Infantry who sustained Japanese machine-gun fire to his upper body and face in New Guinea. Eventually admitted to the care of Archibald McIndoe in 1943, this Australian soldier appears to have set a unique precedent of holding the most appointments on McIndoe's operating table. However, his recorded status of being a member of the Guinea Pig Club, as recorded on the East Grinstead Museum data must be considered conflicting to the rules of club membership.[54]

7

Paragraph **7** of the Minutes of the Guinea Pig Clubs General Meeting in July 1947 states. 'Full membership of the club is to continue to be limited to the categories already laid down, namely: Aircrew patients of the Queen Victoria Hospital, East Grinstead, with the addition of a strictly limited numbers of other Air Force Personnel who could benefit by or benefit from membership.'

0

Another blank within the Hospital records and the register of Guinea Pig Club members relates to the name P. Pereuse. This name has a high probability of being the French airman, Pierre Pereuse. He obtained his pilot's licence in November 1939. Arriving in England in July 1940, he enlisted into the Free French Air Forces. Promoted to lieutenant-colonel in 1943. Pierre de Saint Pereuse became victim to a crash on 15 July 1943 when he was a passenger in a six-seat, twin-engine Caudron Goeland aircraft of the French air liaison group, piloted by Lieutenant Marcel Lebois. He

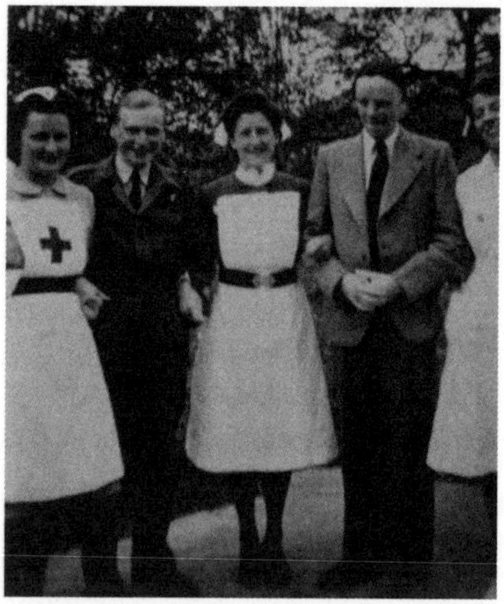

Sid McQuillan standing in uniform with nursing staff and one other Guinea Pig in the grounds at the East Grinstead Hospital. McIndoe challenged some service rules which he felt were unsuited to the Guinea Pigs. McIndoe fought for their right to wear their issued uniforms whenever they chose.

made a forced landing in Algeria and despite his injuries, travelled some distance to seek help for the two survivors. The pilot died that same day. Pereuse was in hospital assumedly in Algeria and thereafter in England at the Queen Victoria Hospital. Pierre Pereuse was later assigned to the French staff facility in Great Britain. The hospital records disclose no detail other than the name. The author's due diligence leads towards the above circumstances, until otherwise advised.

4 Between 1942 and 1946 the **4** burn treatment centres at Halton, Ely, Rauceby and Cosford increased bed capacity from **12** to **14** beds each.

100–130 The annual turnover of patients at each of the **4** centres was between **100** to **130** patients at each facility.

8 The mortality average of admitted patients per annum from the turnover statistic at the **4** burn centre establishments was **8** per cent.[55]

1 In July 1944, a circular letter to all Canadian Air Force units advised them that all cases involving burns, facial injuries, mandibular, maxillary and nasal fractures, as well as all other cases requiring plastic surgery, were to be referred to the new Canadian Wing at the Queen Victoria Hospital in East Grinstead. Assurance was given that cooperation in evacuating injured aircrew by air direct to Gatwick, the airfield nearest to the hospital would be facilitated.

1 A Royal Canadian Air Force film unit arrived at East Grinstead in 1944. In unison with the Canadian National Film Board, they filmed Canadian airmen patients creating a title, 'New Faces Come Back'. Guinea Pig Jack Allaway, despite being British, featured prominently in the fictionalised production.

3 On 12 July 1944, at 7.22am, a German V1 flying bomb fell onto East Grinstead causing three deaths and injuring many others. The bomb landed in close proximity to the Whitehall, adding to the grief which was still present from the cinema bombing. The **3** civilian casualties were George Edwards, James Potten, and Ernest Russell, an Air Raid Precautions officer. The flying bomb had been seen to the south-east of East Grinstead by fighter pilots, Flight Sergeants Langley and Bosley. They fired bursts of gunfire into the bomb which caught fire and fell into the middle of East Grinstead. Within hours of this incident the King and Queen visited the town. They visited the local *Courier* newspaper office which was being used as the incident post at that time. The local newspaper reported: 'The robot had been shot down and diverted by a fighter who was attempting to bring it down in open country and he was afterwards so distressed that he drove specially into East Grinstead to apologise for any damage that had been caused.'[56] The majority of the **41** injured in this incident were treated at the Queen Victoria Hospital.

71

Dutch, Polish, Canadian, Australian, New Zealand and British fighter pilots destroyed **71** V1 flying bombs, commonly called Doodlebugs in the skies over Sussex and Kent on 12 July 1944. The summer onslaught of the jet-propelled pilotless flying bombs upon South-east England and London was relentless. Patients and staff at the Queen Victoria Hospital frequently heard the recognisable sound of the engines as they traversed the skies. Safety was assured until the engine stopped and it plummeted to explode wherever that may have been.[57]

1

The artist Anna Zinkeisen enrolled as an auxiliary nurse and in 1941 she also undertook war artist work for St John's Ambulance Brigade. later specialising in pathological and clinical drawing. She worked in the casualty ward at St Mary's Hospital, Paddington and in 1944 painted and depicted McIndoe operating at the Queen Victoria Hospital in East Grinstead. This painting is now within the collection of the Imperial War Museum, London.

116

The Canadian Wing at East Grinstead Hospital treated **76** Canadian patients, **32** British patients and **8** Allied servicemen of other nationalities between July 1944 and September 1945.[58] The Canadian Wing at East Grinstead in conjunction with the army neurological and plastic surgery hospital at Basingstoke were considered as special treatment centres for plastic surgery. Personnel from all three services could be admitted to either centre.[59] This might well provide an understanding of the patient mix whereby some casualties other than airmen were regarded as Guinea Pig Club members in the latter war years.[60]

1945

One of the difficulties at the Queen Victoria Hospital was the rehabilitation of long-term patients. Meetings in 1945 were arranged between representatives of the hospital welfare committee, the

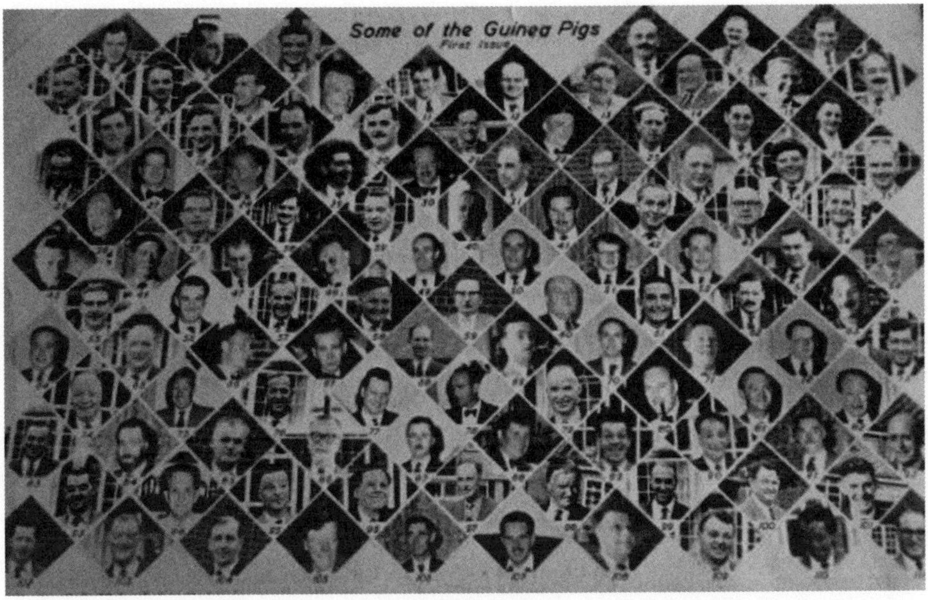

The Guinea Pig newsletter published a request for images of club members. A collage photograph was created and sent to the contributors.

Royal Air Force Benevolent Fund, the British Red Cross Society and the Royal Air Force Rehabilitation Department in order to try and co-ordinate the granting of resettlement allowances. Archibald McIndoe succeeding in persuading authorities to defer discharge from military services employment of these long-term patients. As a full extension of the Queen Victoria Hospital facilities, the Canadian wing managed their long-term patients interests independently. The welfare secretary at the hospital was Ann Newall.

20 It took **20** months following a flying accident for Jack Perry when his heavy bomber exploded on 31 August 1944, before he entered the Queen Victoria Hospital in 1946. He received **14** operations at East Grinstead. The journey to meet Archibald McIndoe was via North Allerton, Rauceley and Marchwood Hospitals.

1 After Alexander Fleming's 1928 discovery of penicillin, research enabled the testing and production of the drug creating the early development of penicillin, developed by Ernest Chain of Russian-German-Jewish descent and the Australian Howard Florey. They were awarded the 1945 Nobel prize for Medicine.[61] In October and November of 1945, the Royal Canadian Air Force was given the task of delivering penicillin into Poland. The medicine, provided by the

Canadian Red Cross was flown to Scotland and then into Warsaw. On board the aircraft was the Canadian Guinea Pig navigator John Harding. He had become a Guinea Pig after an accident in an aircraft that crashed taking off in January 1945. The burn injuries he sustained had been operated upon twice at the Queen Victoria Hospital in February that year.

1

A Royal Navy Reserve sailor who occupied a bed in Ward Three in 1945 was Leslie Jago who had served on the Arctic Murmansk convoys. He required surgery on his hands and feet, assumed to be for frostbite injuries. The work by the surgeons was forever appreciated and although not a Guinea Pig he supported and attended many reunions as an official friend of the Guinea Pig Club.[62]

£3,000

A gift of **£3,000** was received in 1946 sent from New Zealand to Captain W. H. Banham, the then secretary superintendent of the Queen Victoria Hospital, East Grinstead. The grant had been approved by the New Zealand Cabinet in recognition of the work done for New Zealand airmen who suffered from burns requiring plastic surgery.[63]

3

Following the Second World War, Gillies, McIndoe and Mowlem remained in the United Kingdom and continued in partnership at 149 Harley Street, whilst still undertaking work at their wartime hospitals.

1946

McIndoe's first marriage had become strained which eventually resulted in an official separation in **1946**. Whilst his wife resided at Chatsworth Court in Kensington, McIndoe's daughters both remained living with him in Sussex. Mabel McIndoe, Archibald's mother also moved to East Grinstead and moved into a property in St Johns Road. His mother was an outstanding artist of repute.

100

The establishment of nurses at the hospital in 1946 was over **100**. Nurses were accommodated in **4** nurses' homes in East Grinstead.

1946

Phillip Barrowman a member of the Royal Air Force Medical Branch arrived at East Grinstead in this year. He was allocated accommodation in Holtye Road and performed liaison duties with medical boards and patient transfers. It is assumed that Archibald McIndoe instigated that the hospital's medical records required the cross indexing of registers for operations and injuries as an important matter. The task took nearly two years to complete.[64]

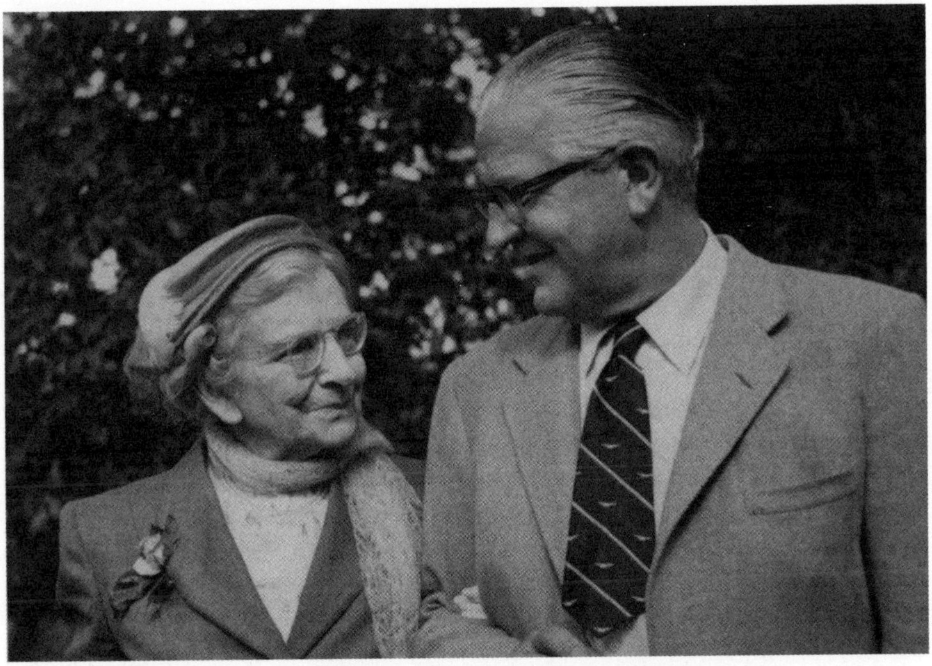

Archibald McIndoe seen wearing his Guinea Pig Club tie with his mother, Mabel McIndoe. An artist of some repute, Mrs McIndoe died at the Queen Victoria Hospital on 18 November 1956, aged **84** years.

Phillip Barrowman later became the official Hospital Medical Records Officer at the Queen Victoria Hospital working with John Myson and Elsie Myson.[65]

The Queen arrived at the Queen Victoria hospital on 25 July 1946 to officially open the 'American Wing'. Mr Clark Minor president of the British War Relief Society represented the American department alongside Mr Harriman the United States Ambassador. Also present were Lord Kindersley the hospitals president, Lord Woolton of the Red Cross with Lords Portal and Tedder of the Royal Air Force. The Queen went to a luncheon with Lord and Lady Kindersley, Lady Louis Mountbatten, Lady Katherine Seymour, Mr & Mrs Edward Blount, Mr Alfred Wagg and Archibald McIndoe.[66]

1947 The Corneo-Plastic Unit and regional eye bank was formed in this year at the Queen Victoria Hospital, thereafter addressing all eye socket surgery and corneal grafts.

1 A 22-seater motor coach, the gift of Lord Nuffield, was presented to East Grinstead Queen Victoria Hospital on New Year's Day 1947.[67]

1947

Archibald McIndoe received his Knighthood in this year.

1948

The Guinea Pig Club's Canadian Wing was officially formed in November of this year. Group Captain Ross Tilley the head of the Canadian Wing at Queen Victoria Hospital became their president. Flying Officer Donald Freeborn who became a Guinea Pig in October 1944 was appointed the new club's secretary. Pilot Officer Paul Weber, a Guinea Pig burned in a crash also in 1944, became the treasurer.

40

A criminal court case involved a Guinea Pig Club imposter. In October 1949, there was a case heard at Gloucestershire Assizes. The defendant was Mr. Reginald Hugh Wadsworth Bundle, who was indicted on **40** counts of passing worthless cheques. Mr. Bundle was a severely disfigured man – the results of burns apparently sustained in an aircraft crash. He admitted the fraud offences with his legal representative mitigating that it was due to Bundle's serious burn injuries, citing that he had undergone **47** operations and was a member of the Guinea Pig Club. The officer in the case, Detective Sergeant Price, from Cirencester, doubted this. He realised that the impact of such a claim could attract a substantial degree of sympathy from the Court. He asked for time to verify the claim made by Mr. Bundle and was granted an adjournment. The case returned to the Assizes on 1 November 1949. Detective Sergeant Price had contacted Sir Archibald McIndoe and presented evidence to the Court that Mr. Bundle was not a member of the Guinea Pig Club.[68]

1953

Sir Archibald McIndoe's divorce from Adonia was finalised in this year. In 1954 he remarried, his second wife being Lady Constance Belchem, a divorcee whom he had known since 1947. Constance McIndoe inevitably attended the annual Guinea Pig Club reunions, supporting Archibald in all respects of his life.

1

John Hunter, the anaesthetist and great friend to Archibald McIndoe who created such friendships with the many Guinea Pig patients he sedated, fell into ill health in 1953. He had been a lifelong sufferer from diabetes. John Hunter was later admitted to the Queen Victoria Hospital and spent his last few days amid the surroundings he had known so well. John having gently applied drowsiness to innumerable patients, succumbed himself and died on 9 August 1953.

1 Mrs M. McIndoe, the mother of Sir Archibald, underwent an eye operation at the Queen Victoria Hospital in November 1956. She also died in the hospital on 18 November, aged 84 years.

1957 The Peanut Club now registered as a charity, declared an objective to purchase equipment for the Queen Victoria Hospital.[69]

1958 Amongst the last patients to join the Guinea Pig Club was Robert George Chitham. He was not an airman but a Medical Officer. He qualified as a doctor in 1953, and enlisted in the Royal Canadian Air Force shortly thereafter, serving as a Station Medical Officer at Grostenquin, north-eastern France. In 1958 two aircraft collided above the airfield where he was based. One engine fell away and crashed into the corridor outside of Robert's office bursting into flames. He was with difficulty able to escape the building, rolling on the ground to extinguish his flaming uniform. The fire spread towards the station nursery and he bravely re-entered the building and went to the nursery, giving instructions to move the cribs and to disconnect the incubators from their oxygen cylinders. Having suffered significant burn injuries, thought to have been life-threatening, and lost some fingers, he was evacuated to a hospital and later transferred to the RAF Hospital at Halton. He eventually arrived at the Queen Victoria Hospital under the care of Sir Archibald McIndoe; his injuries required a three-year medical recovery in Sussex.[70]

5 As 1960 commenced, the reputation of the Queen Victoria Hospital had seemingly reached its pinnacle. The gift of the British War Relief Society of America had created the American Wing which had established an additional **5** theatres.[71] Additionally, Sir Archibald McIndoe had been engaged in planning for the establishment of a Research Unit at East Grinstead with Mr and Mrs Blond who provided a significant donation. The Blond McIndoe Centre for Medical Research at East Grinstead opened in 1960. Sir Archibald McIndoe was by then Vice-President of the Royal College of Surgeons.

3 The hospital has the unique record in that the chiefs of its **3** major surgical departments – Archibald McIndoe, plastic surgery, Benjamin Rycroft, cornea-plastic surgery and Terence Ward, oral surgery – were all honoured with knighthoods.

1 A public bench was presented by East Grinstead Council to the Queen Victoria Hospital Guinea Pig Club. A large engraved plaque

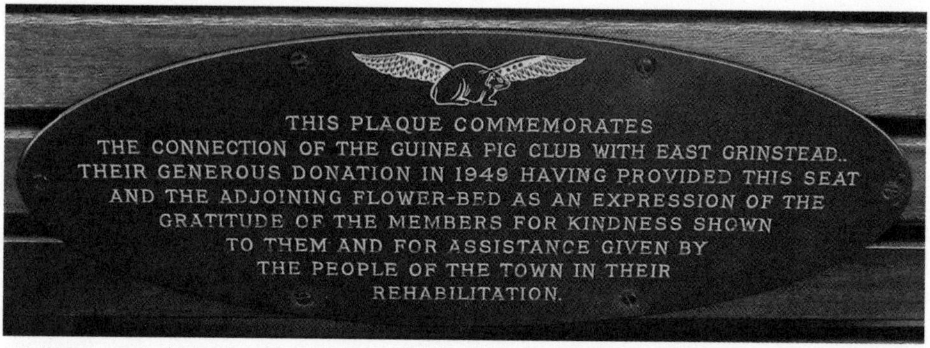
THIS PLAQUE COMMEMORATES
THE CONNECTION OF THE GUINEA PIG CLUB WITH EAST GRINSTEAD.
THEIR GENEROUS DONATION IN 1949 HAVING PROVIDED THIS SEAT
AND THE ADJOINING FLOWER-BED AS AN EXPRESSION OF THE
GRATITUDE OF THE MEMBERS FOR KINDNESS SHOWN
TO THEM AND FOR ASSISTANCE GIVEN BY
THE PEOPLE OF THE TOWN IN THEIR
REHABILITATION.

The Guinea Pig Club presented a public bench to the people of East Grinstead. The seat displays an engraved plaque with the crest of the club and words of gratitude to the people of East Grinstead. The seat can be found near to the statue of Sir Archibald McIndoe outside Sackville College. The plaque is a meaningful statement of the heartfelt appreciation of readily accepting injured airmen, regardless of their disfigurement, in East Grinstead.

expressed the gratitude of the people of East Grinstead and the seat was placed for public use in the town.

1960

By early 1960, Sir Archibald McIndoe's heart and health were failing. Despite this, he put himself forward for election to President of the Royal College of Surgeons of England. Having attended the Royal College of Surgeons Council annual dinner on 11 April 1960, McIndoe returned to his accommodation in London. He died whilst sleeping in the early hours of 12 April, knowing that his election as President of the College was a certainty.

1

1 edition of the Guinea Pig magazine has a blank front cover. This was the edition which followed the news of McIndoe's death. The Royal College of Surgeons of England immediately wrote in memoriam whereby his skills as both surgeon and man were lauded in that edition.

1

His Royal Highness, Prince Philip, Duke of Edinburgh, having accepted the invitation to act as the president of the Guinea Pig Club by Lady McIndoe, was presented with his badge of office. His Golden Guinea Pig badge was presented by the Chairman of the club, Tom Gleave at an informal reception on 22 November 1960.

6

The modern Queen Victoria Hospital has **6** locations with identities relevant to the Second World War. The history of the hospital is celebrated by the Peanut Ward, Ross Tilley Ward, McIndoe's Meeting Room, Spitfire Restaurant, Hurricane Café and the Lancaster Lounge.

1962 The year in which the McIndoe lecture was founded. It was achieved with the proceeds of an appeal sponsored by the Royal Air Force Association in memory of Sir Archibald McIndoe. It became a bi-annual lecture on plastic surgery, or another allied subject. The lecturer is nominated by the College and President along with the Honorary Secretary of the British Association of Plastic Surgeons. A large round cast commemorative medal is presented to each lecturer which is embellished with the Guinea Pig Club badge.

1963 In 1963, the Queen Victoria Hospital's centenary year, Her Majesty Queen Elizabeth laid the foundation stone of the new McIndoe Burns Centre. Today, those facilities and the legacy of the Guinea Pig Club ensures the Queen Victoria Hospital is an internationally renowned specialist centre for reconstructive surgery.

1965 On 5 July 1965 Princess Marina, Duchess of Kent opened the Sterile Burns Centre at the Queen Victoria Hospital. The Guinea Pig Club was represented by the presence of Henry Standen, Reg Hyde and Hugh Parratt.

Chapter 3

The Guinea Pigs in Wartime

1 Polish pilot Jerzy Glebocki most likely suffered the first injuries sustained by any Guinea Pig in the Second World War. During the invasion of Poland in September 1939, Luftwaffe bombing inflicted facial lacerations from glass or other debris upon him as bombs exploded in close proximity to his motor car. Initial medical treatment in a Polish hospital was temporary as he escaped his country to reach England and fly within Bomber Command. It was **5** years after his injuries, in early 1945 that his old scarring was operated upon at East Grinstead.[1]

1,127 The Battle of France took place between 3 September 1939 and 24 June 1940. The Royal Air Force suffered **1,127** airmen shot down, parachuted out of an aircraft or crash landing. Alan Kenneth Summerson was one of these and would become a member of the Guinea Pig Club. On 14 May 1940, he was a Leading Aircraftsman, Air Gunner flying in a Battle light bomber attacking pontoon bridges during the failed attempts to thwart the German advance into France. Shot down in flames, the aircraft crashed at Raucourt-et-flaba in the Ardennes. Summerson had a bullet wound to his leg and had been thrown clear from the aircraft. His pilot and observer were trapped and he attempted a rescue which prove impossible. His attempts caused burn injuries and he was losing blood. Suffering temporary blindness from his facial burns he sought refuge as best he could. Once he gained some sight, he set off and came to the French lines where he was taken to Verdun hospital. He was treated for injuries to his hands, face, back and right leg. Moves to Roanne and then Marseille hospitals were followed by repatriation to the Queen Victoria Hospital in the spring of 1941. The French Government later recognised his heroic efforts by awarding him the Medaille Militaire and Cross de Guerre.[2] It appears that Alan Summerson is the only Guinea Pig to have been awarded that combination of French medals.

4 On 24 May 1940, Herbert Benjamin Bell-Syer was flying one of **4** Hurricanes when they engaged a large force of Luftwaffe aircraft over Amiens, France. Bell-Syer was shot down and last seen descending on a parachute. Nothing further was heard of him until the first week of June 1940 when he was located in a hospital at Grand Luce, in the region of Pays de la Loire in north-western France. He was badly injured, with burns to his face and head, temporarily blinded and also suffering from shrapnel wounds in one of his legs.[3] After the capitulation of France, he was fortunate to receive a medical repatriation due to his burn injuries. At a date unknown he was admitted to the Queen Victoria Hospital.[4] His treatment was apparently immediate and it appears from official records of flying that he returned to fly on a non-operational footing by joining the Armament Testing Squadron at Boscombe Down. Around this time his father Squadron Leader Russel Bell-Syer's untimely death was reported in several newspapers. He had collapsed and died while flying as a passenger. At the time of his death, he was officer commanding at a Lincolnshire station.[5] His son Herbert Bell-Syer is undoubtably an entitled member of the Guinea Pig Club but he is not recorded on any roll of honour.

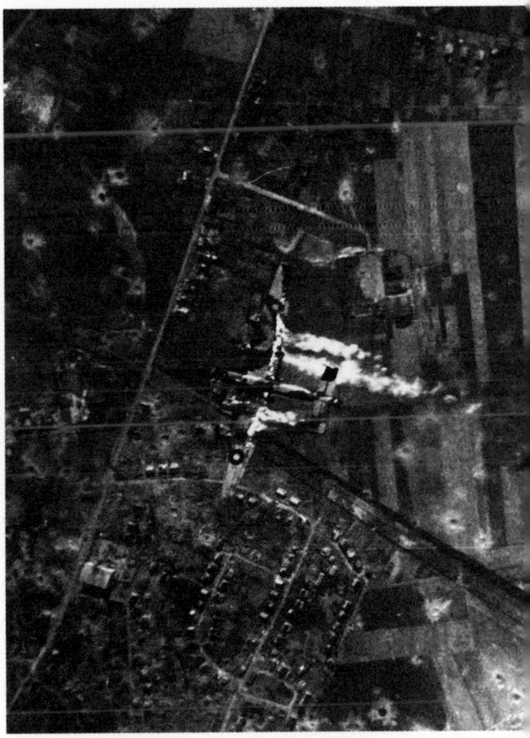

A burning Halifax heavy bomber flying over occupied territory. The wing fuel tanks ablaze, the fate of the crew is unknown.

0 The name A. Deniall is recorded upon the register of Guinea Pigs which hangs as the memorial board in the Queen Victoria Hospital. However, in respect of the name upon the memorial board, no additional detail is known. Archibald McIndoe made passing reference to a French pilot, Andre Deniau, in one of his post-war newsletters. It is the author's perception that these details relate to Adjutant Pilot Deniel who flew during the Battle of France in fighter aircraft within the French GC

111/36 squadron. Undoubtably this pilot received medical treatment by Archibald McIndoe and the differing spelling of the names is no doubt a simple error. A high probability exists that this French pilot was an early Guinea Pig.[6]

1,497

The exponential growth of Bomber Command, in particular crews in training, suffered many accidents creating many burn patients. The heavy bomber aircraft created opportunities for multiple burn casualties in one aircraft. In 1944, the statistics indicate a casualty figure of **1,497** men who had suffered significant burns that year.[7]

1,425

An almost identical statistic exists as evidenced by the RAF Medical Services Officer, Group Captain S. C. Rexford Welch. He discloses the total number of airmen treated during the war who endured burn injuries to their arms and hands having been **1,425**.[8] It has to be assumed this figure originates from records across the primary burn units within the Royal Air Force hospitals.

1

Royal Air Force Station Medical Officers issued every member of aircrew with a small personal first aid pack. It was well devised, the whole pack being able to be ripped open diagonally in a moment. Aircrew burn injuries needed to be treated at the earliest moment possible to reduce infection.

1,300

The exact number of cases treated by the various burn centres and other units over the war years is impossible to deduce, particularly as many of the cases involved multiple injuries and were often under the care of several specialists. The following figure established by Squadron Leader Rexford-Welch indicates the numbers of Royal Air Force casualty cases which passed through the East Grinstead Queen Victoria Hospital, from its commencement until 1945 reached a total of more than **1,300** cases where burns were treated.[9]

825

Facial injuries, specifically sustained by burns between 1939 and 1945 were, according to Squadron Leader Rexford Welch, marginally over **800**. The statistics are quantified by Rexford Welch as relating to 'Home Force' personnel only. This has to be interpreted as men operating from within the United Kingdon.

3

In 1941, **3** meals of high protein content were being advocated for burns cases. In 1942, high-protein diets became officially recognised as beneficial. Instructions were delivered to all RAF hospitals including the Queen Victoria Hospital to deliver as advocated.[10]

1

Only **1** Guinea Pig Club airman was awarded the Military Medal. Richard Pape was shot down in September 1941. His aircraft crashed near Hengalo in the eastern part of the Netherlands. He escaped the scene and was assisted by the Dutch resistance. During his evasion he was arrested by the Gestapo. Richard escaped from custody only to be recaptured once again. This time he was brutally interrogated before being sent to a prison camp. After an orchestrated medical repatriation to Britain which he ingeniously devised himself, he recuperated and returned to service. He was posted to retrain with flying duties on the Isle of Man where he became hospitalised due to an accident on a motorcycle. His injuries are ill defined however he was subsequently taken to Sussex where two operations were undertaken at the Queen Victoria Hospital in February 1946. His Military Medal was published in *The London Gazette* on 2 September 1947. Richard Pape became a popular individual with McIndoe and his family.[11] The Military Medal was predominantly an Army award and regarded as a prestigious award to an airman. Such awards inevitably relate to escape and evasion activities.

8

The number of Guinea Pigs admitted having sustained injuries in motorcycle accidents.

42

Josef Biel, another Polish pilot, had initially flown against the Luftwaffe when his country was invaded. He like so many, escaped and made his way to Britain via Romania, Turkey and France before flying for the RAF. He qualified as a Spitfire pilot and over Holland, on 8 August 1941, he suffered burn injuries to his face and hands as his aircraft exploded in flames. Escaping by parachute, he became a prisoner of war. Biel spent **42** months as a prisoner before arriving at East Grinstead in 1945. Fellow Polish pilot Brunon Bilinski who had been shot down on 8 November 1941, described a meeting with Biel in Stalag VIIIB prison camp at Lamsdorf: 'In February 1942, Josef Biel arrived, who had been sent from a German hospital, where they had somewhat repaired his burnt face. Oh, horror I didn't recognise him at all, I felt completely crushed when standing in front of me, he said: "Bruno, don't you recognise me. It's me, Josef Biel". In front of me stood a man with a terribly burned face without hair or eyebrows, a nose like a giant crackling and burnt ears. What could I say to him. However, I quickly replied: "Oh Josef of course" … He did not shake my hand in greeting, because both of his hands were terribly burned. The stench of burned flesh could still be felt around him.'[12] Whilst at East Grinstead Hospital, Guinea

Pig Josef Biel wrote to a Miss Stanford in Fulham. He wrote about the nine operations he received at the Hospital, as well as his long road back to health. The following are relevant extracts providing an insight to the medical treatment endured.

5.8.45 Last week I have been in East Grinstead and I had an interview with my doctor and on the 3 September I am going to his hospital for my beauty treatment.

10.9.45 I am in the hospital already. I am well and in good spirits, waiting for my beauty treatment. I expected to have an operation last week but it has been postponed indefinitely as they are reorganising hospital … it is very nice here and everybody is very kind to me. The people in the town are very hospitable so I go out practically every night.

23.8.46 The head surgeon Mr McIndoe is at present operating in Sweden so I was examined this morning by Squadron Leader Moor and told that I shall be operated upon on Tuesday. I don't know yet who will be operating on me but most probably Squadron Leader Moor or a Polish doctor. They are both very good. The Polish doctor who is at present sick saw me last night, we had a long talk, and he examined me and said that he will fix me properly. They are going to lift up my both eyelids at the same time so I shall be blind for about four or five days.

8.9.46 My left eye is still covered and my right eye doesn't feel too comfortable yet but I can read a bit. Anyhow I am very pleased to tell you that my operation was successful and at last I am able to close my eyes properly. My nose has healed nicely and the left hand is doing quite well. I had comparatively a very easy time after operation though I was blind for nine days … A Polish surgeon operated on me; he took two pieces of skin from behind my ears and grafted them under the eyes; the grafted skin has taken nicely and it looks quite nice already. The eyelids have perfect shape again. They opened my right nostril and done a L-plastic on my left hand. I have to say that I am very pleased with his work on me. He says that I shall be a smart looking boy when he finishes with me.

10.9.46 I had a letter from my sister today informing me that the life of my mother is in real danger … I am pleased to tell you that my operation was successful and that I can close my eyes properly. Since yesterday my eyes are uncovered and I have just a small dressing. My hand is doing well too and I started exercise today.

7.10.46 I have just arrived to hospital from my leave and I feel tired after a long journey except that I am rather busy preparing things as I am having another operation tomorrow. This time I shall get a pair of eyebrows so I shall be blind for about a week … In case you would like to come down here, you can visit me any day on the afternoon. I am in Canadian Wing.

18.10.46 I am also glad to tell you that my operation was a success and the new eyebrows look quite nice; they have changed my appearance greatly.

3.11.46 I had to leave hospital a bit earlier than I ought to and my right eyebrow is not doing too well; it got a bit septic; the left one looks very nice. I do hope that the right one will improve soon.

9.1.47 I am very sorry for not having written to you in so long but my eyes were very bad and for about two weeks I hardly could see. I have to tell you (to avoid a lecture on eyesight) that my eyes went bad as a result of my accident in the Air Force, and the eye-specialist told me that this may happen from time to time … At last I am on unpaid leave from the Air Force but I have to sign to the Resettlement Corps.

4.7.47 I have been in hospital since the end of May when my eyes went bad. Being here I have decided to finish my beauty treatment and I have had two operations already; both of them were successful. By the end of next week, I am expecting to leave the hospital for ten days leave and by the end of this month I shall have my last operation.

7.8.47 I have been in hospital since 28 July and that I have had my operation on July 30. This time they grafted one piece of my ear on the right side of my nose but I nearly lost the graft as the wound was bleeding for four days. Using all sorts of tricks my doctor won the battle for the nose which now looks quite nice.

24.1.48 I left hospital on the 10 Jan and had a week rest in Lincoln. I spent 8 weeks in hospital and had one operation which was successful though after that operation I was feeling very badly; I never felt worse and I thought I was going to leave this earthly sphere of misery to start another life. Anyway, I survived and I have to go to East Grinstead once more in summertime. I spent Xmas in hospital and had quite nice time under the circumstances; plenty of food and drink and Sir Archibald McIndoe done all the carving for us with an expert hand; he also dined with us and after dinner he played the piano for us. Most of the time at Xmas I spent in a wheelchair but on New Years eve I went out as I wanted to get drunk.

1.2.48 The reason for me being in a wheelchair was that they took skin from my leg so I couldn't walk for about two weeks as that kind of thing is very painful.

28.7.48 I am in the hospital again to complete my beauty treatment … I am having my operation tomorrow morning.

12.2.49 Last Thursday I had my last operation this was definitely my last one and next week I shall be out of hospital for good so I won't be able to see your friend here … I am going to my station to be invalided out and then I shall be looking to earn my living. I have a job in Birmingham to go to but I don't think I can cope with it at present as my left hand is of not much use since I had a new graft put on it. I shall find a big improvement after two or three months. I was absolutely mad two weeks ago as they wanted to discharge me without giving me invaliding board anyway I managed to persuade them but I am still anticipating trouble.

16.3.49 My eyes are not troubling me at present. I have finished my treatment at East Grinstead completely and I am a civilian already.

12.9.49 So your friend is a 'friend of Guinea Pigs' I seem to know her name … I enjoyed the Guinea Pig dance as well as the Annual Dinner in spite of the fact that I had a headache for three days after these celebrations as I drunk more than ever … I have another surprise

> for you. I am about to be engaged to a girl who was nursing me in East Grinstead. Her name is Betty as well, and she is now a sister in East Grinstead.[13]

Josef Biel received the Polish Cross of Valour. He married the East Grinstead nursing sister only identified as Betty and celebrated his marriage with a son and daughter.

101

Maurice Mounsdon, one of the Battle of Britain fighter pilots and subsequent Guinea Pig club members, lived to reach the age of **101**. He flew as a Hurricane pilot in 1940, based at North Weald. He was successful in combat against the Luftwaffe securing two confirmed kills, two probable, and two damaged during the Battle of Britain. He was shot down whilst attacking enemy bombers flying over Colchester, Essex on 31 August 1940. The combat saw his Hurricane aircraft burst into flames causing him injuries before he managed to escape by parachute. He landed near the village of Great Easter and was given help by local villagers. He spent time at the Black Notley Sanatorium hospital in Braintree Essex before admission into the care of Archibald McIndoe on 8 January 1941. Five operations were undertaken on his injuries at the Queen Victoria Hospital. His notable injuries were multiple burns to his face, hands, legs and thigh. In addition, the Luftwaffe fighter gunfire which shot his aircraft down also penetrated his left thigh. Maurice recovered sufficiently to remain in service and immediately after the war, he served in the Disarmament Wing tasked with searching throughout Germany for intelligence of advanced rocket weaponry.[14]

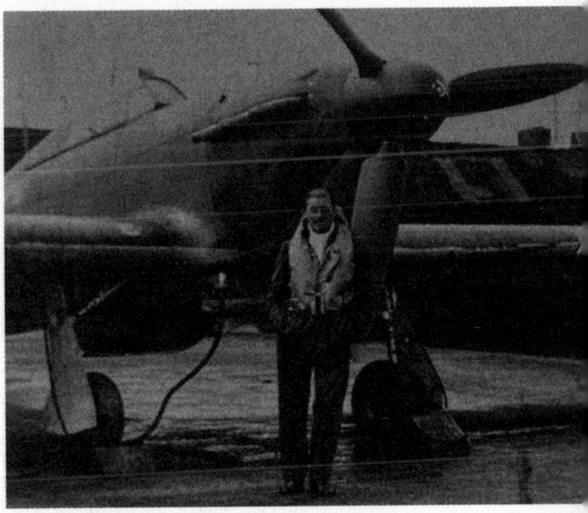

Maurice Mounsdon standing with his Hurricane which is positioned in a sandbag blast pen designed to prevent damage from enemy bombs.

1

1 Guinea Pig Club member was recommended to be awarded the highly esteemed, Medal of the Order of the British Empire for Gallantry. However, within weeks of the award notification, the King instituted the Order of the British Empire for Gallantry medal, which was to be replaced by the George Cross.[15] The George Cross was effectively a response to the changing nature of the Second World War. King George VI announced it would recognise supreme gallantry away from the heat of battle and in recognising civilian situations of bravery. It was on 11 March 1940, when Flying Officer Anthony Henry Hamilton Tollemache, flying his Bristol Blenheim, crashed while attempting to land at Manston, Kent. Flying Officer Tollemache was thrown clear of the wreckage, His air gunner was able to escape without difficulty but realising that his passenger Second Lieutenant Sperling was still in the aircraft. Tollemache, with complete disregard of the intense conflagration and the explosion of small arms ammunition, endeavoured to break through the forward hatch and effect a rescue. He persisted in this gallant attempt until driven off with his clothes blazing. His efforts had resulted in injuries which nearly cost him his life. His efforts were in vain, however, as sadly Sperling had died in the flames. Anthony Tollemache suffered significant and deep burns in the incident. A local farmer arrived and carried the two surviving airmen to Manston airfield where Tollemache was initially treated by Dr Attwood the station medical officer. Fearing for his patient's life, Tollemache was immediately sent to Chatham Naval Hospital where the symptoms of his severe burns were stabilised. Tollemache arrived at the Queen Victoria Hospital on 17 May 1940. He underwent four surgeries for his wounds. Flying Officer Tollemache is the only Guinea Pig Club member to carry the title of GC (George Cross) after his name. The Investiture of his George Cross took place in September 1941 by King George VI, at Buckingham Palace.[16]

5

On 10 May 1940, Sergeant Kenneth Norman Varwell Townsend gained the status of an 'Ace' by shooting down **5** enemy aircraft. One incident remarkably saw him observing one of his damaged victim's aircraft land at the grass airfield at St Quentin airfield, north of Paris. Townsend also landed and set off chasing the fleeing enemy bomber crew. With the help of the French stationed at the airfield, all of the Luftwaffe crew were successfully captured.[17] On 11 May Townsend had success again against another Luftwaffe bomber which was unconfirmed but damaged. He was immediately awarded the Distinguished Flying Medal for such outstanding flying.[18] However, the following day, 12 May, he was shot down flying his Hurricane over Belgium. Townsend had sustained shrapnel injuries before his aircraft burst into flames. Despite his burns and other injuries, he successfully bailed out over Lens-Saint-Servais, Belgium and was captured on landing west of Tourinne. His injuries received medical attention in both Belgium and Germany. Thereafter he endured four years in a prisoner of war camp. Kenneth Townsend was repatriated on the SS *Gripsholm* arriving in England on 16 September 1944. He was admitted to the East Grinstead hospital. The dates and surgery by Archibald McIndoe are unknown but undoubtedly it related to scar injury treatment to his old burns. Kenneth Townsend became a Guinea Pig several years after his wounds had been inflicted. He is undoubtably the only Guinea Pig pilot who personally captured the crew of an enemy aircraft he had shot down in battle over France.[19]

13 The repatriation of injured prisoners of war only became a consideration if the German forces assumed the man's injuries were such that he no longer posed a threat to Nazi Germany. These identified prisoners were held in special Heilag or Heimkehrerlager camps. There were approximately **13** Heilags known to exist. The Red Cross engaged in the repatriation of pilots and airmen. Once repatriated they were inevitably distributed within the primary RAF hospitals with only a small percentage being treated by Archibald McIndoe.

3 Spitfire pilot Eric Lock was the only Guinea Pig to be presented with **3** gallantry awards during one Investiture conducted by the King at Buckingham Palace. Pilot Officer Eric Lock's gallantry is best understood by referencing the official publications of his awards by the Air Ministry. He was first awarded the Distinguished Flying Cross on 1 October 1940. 'This officer has destroyed nine enemy aircraft, eight of these within a period of one week. He has displayed great vigour and determination in pressing home his attacks.' The Air Ministry further announced on 22 October 1940 that he had been awarded a Bar to the Distinguished Flying Cross. 'In September, 1940, whilst engaged on a patrol over the Dover area, Pilot Officer Lock engaged three Heinkel 113's one of which he shot down into the sea. Immediately afterwards he engaged a Henschel Hs 126 and destroyed it. He has displayed great courage in the face of heavy odds, and his skill and coolness in combat have enabled him to destroy fifteen enemy aircraft within a period of nineteen days.' The Air Ministry further announced on 17 December, 1940, that Eric Lock was appointed a Companion of the Distinguished Service Order. 'This officer has shown exceptional keenness and courage in his attacks against the enemy. In November, 1940, whilst engaged with his squadron in attacking a superior number of enemy forces, he destroyed two Messerschmitt 109's, thus bringing his total to at least twenty-two. His magnificent fighting spirit and personal example have been in the highest traditions of the service.' It was on 8 November 1940 over Dungeness when he sustained severe wounds in both legs and his left arm and force-landed near Manston. He was taken to Ipswich Hospital before arriving at Halton where Archibald McIndoe required him to be taken to East Grinstead. At the Queen Victoria Hospital, he underwent fifteen operations. On 1 April 1941 he attended the Buckingham Palace investiture. In June 1941 he climbed back into the cockpit of a Spitfire but on 3 August 1941 he failed to return from operations over Calais France. In unknown circumstances made worse by the fact that his body was never located, Eric Lock is remembered as a most distinguished member of the Guinea Pig Club.[20]

3

Almost on the eve of 1941, John Malcolm Poole was on a cross-country flying exercise with his crew in a Blenheim bomber when they were shot down by a Luftwaffe intruder. John Poole was taken to the Royal Air Force Hospital Ely, before being transferred to East Grinstead on 11 January. He spent a year in the hospital enduring **3** operations upon his fractured jaw and burn injuries. He was the sole survivor of his crew.[21]

14

John G. E. Munt was flying from Thorney Island on the Sussex Coast in 1941. On 30 March 1941, his crew and two other crews all flying Blenheim light bombers were tasked with attacking an enemy convoy of shipping off the French Coast at Calais. As they crossed the English Channel, the enemy ships were sighted but unexpectedly it was being protected by Luftwaffe fighter aircraft. Despite the odds of success, the attack was pressed home, but as they did so, Munt's Blenheim was singled out for a series of individual attacks by the enemy fighters. He was in the Blenheim's air gunner's turret when enemy cannon shells raked along the fuselage just below his turret. His lower body was in line of the gunfire which tore into his buttocks, legs and feet.[22] Only when halfway across the Channel and limping back towards Kent did two Spitfire pilots provide any safety. One of the Spitfires was being flown by Jackie Mann who directed the Blenheim towards Hawkinge airfield. By a strange coincidence, Mann was also destined to become a Guinea Pig with injuries he sustained in his own Spitfire, four days after these events. The Blenheim belly-landed on the edge of Hawkinge airfield. The aircraft was all but destroyed. Munt was lifted out through the escape hatch and taken to the hospital in Folkestone. **14** days later, he was transferred to the Queen Victoria Hospital. Inexplicably Jackie Mann and John Munt were admitted to the care of Archibald McIndoe on that same day, 14 April 1941. The hospital records for John Munt are sparse. For Jackie Mann, his injuries are defined as burns to his face and legs in addition to a wound sustained by enemy gunfire into his left elbow. At a date unknown, John was later invalided out of military service whilst Jackie Mann recovered sufficiently to be assessed as fit to fly aircraft for ferrying duties sometime in 1942.

1 Canadian pilot Clark Chater is the only known member of the Guinea Pig Club who joined whilst flying an aircraft without an engine. He had been posted to serve in England as a flying instructor on gliders and held the rank of Pilot Officer, the circumstances of his accident are unknown. The injuries sustained required nine months' residency at the Queen Victoria hospital in 1942. Clark Chater became a supporter of the Canadian Wing of the Guinea Pig Club in his home country, and was registered as a member until 1977.

3 Guinea Pig Farnham King crashed in a Whitley bomber on 23 March 1941. He was practising circuits and landings at Abingdon in Oxfordshire. A heavy touchdown landing resulted in the aircraft bouncing back into the air and as the pilot commenced to gain height, a wing clipped a tree causing a crash into Wootton Road where it burst into flames. Farnham King survived with burns and other injuries which saw him receive treatment in **3** hospitals. It was whilst he was a patient at the Royal Air Force Hospital Halton that he was identified as a patient for Archibald McIndoe. He arrived at East Grinstead on 2 October 1941. Farnham King's broken leg complications resulted in his leg being in a plaster cast for two years, a most unusual occurrence.[23]

5 The Battle of Britain Spitfire pilot William Anderson Douglas returned to operations within **5** months of injuries inflicted upon him on 23 June 1941. He was near Calais, flying an operation involving several squadrons of fighters covering a small force of light bombers acting as bait for the enemy fighters to attack. William Douglas entered into combat with the Luftwaffe fighters which resulted in him sustaining wounds inflicted by return cannon fire. Shells had struck his aircraft and exploded sending shrapnel into his cockpit. Fortunate to escape, he was able to fly back to

England. After initial medical attention to his injuries, Douglas was transported to the East Grinstead Hospital where the first of three operations commenced upon the wounds to both his legs and one arm. It appears that nerve damage surgery, most likely to his arm took place sometime later at the Wingfield-Norris Orthopaedic Hospital in Oxford. In November 1941, just **5** months after his injuries, Douglas returned to operational flying. In April 1942, he was posted overseas to the besieged island of Malta. On 11 May 1942, in a crowded sky, Douglas collided with another Spitfire during the aerial interception of enemy bombers. Both pilots escaped by parachute and were rescued. William Douglas went on to claim three enemy aircraft shot down before he returned to the United Kingdom for rest and instructional flying. This Guinea Pig Club member was recommended for the Distinguished Flying Cross in December 1942. It is a rare example of gallant flying post-surgery and recovery. William Douglas also gained a 'Bar' signifying a further Distinguished Flying Cross awarded to him in 1944. He was an exceptional survivor who eventually retired as an 'Ace status' pilot Guinea Pig in the rank of Wing Commander.[24]

1 One street name in Paris, Rue Du Commandant-Schloesing, is dedicated to the French Guinea Pig club member Captain Jacques-Henri Schloesing. He was originally shot down above the Somme in his Spitfire and escaped by parachute landing at Campigneulle on 13 February 1943. Badly injured, he made a good escape before being hidden by members of the French Resistance. The resistance network nursed him to a level of fitness whereby he was capable of escaping back to England by the Comet escape line into Spain and Gibraltar. Schloesing crossed the Pyrenees with Jean-François Nothomb[25] in company with a Belgian and four French airmen. Their mountain guide was the renowned Florentino who took numerous evaders over the mountains.[26] Jacques-Henri Schloesing returned to England by aircraft on 8 May 1943. Arriving in London, he was interviewed for intelligence on 9 May 1943. His burn injuries and scaring were finally treated by Archibald McIndoe. The admission date into East Grinstead is unknown, however ten operations were undertaken. He was awarded the Distinguished Flying Cross on 4 August 1943, along with the French Legion of Honour and Croix de Guerre. He took to the skies once more a year later, in May 1944 and participated in the Normandy landings on 6 June 1944. When providing air support to the troops in the invasion of France he was shot down and killed over the Foret de Bray on 26 August

1944. He was buried in the town of Beauvoir-en-Lyon, Normandy. On 27 November 1964, the Rue des Reservoirs, in the 16th arrondissement of Paris, was renamed Rue du Commandant-Schloesing in his honour. The Rolls Royce engine of his Spitfire PL395 was found and excavated in 1983. It is now preserved and on display at the Resistance Museum in Forges-les-Eaux.

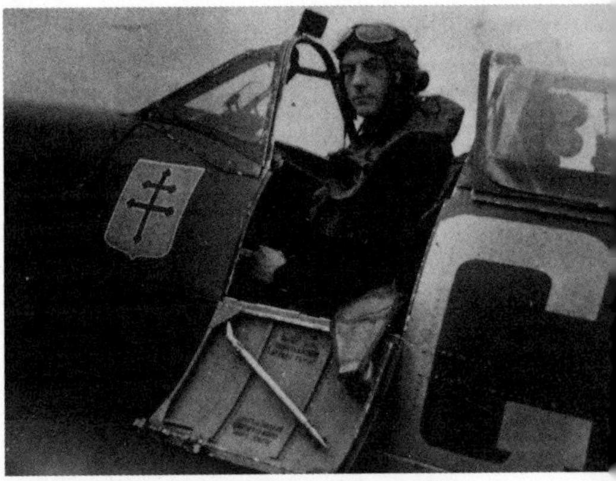

The French Guinea Pig club member Captain Jacques-Henri Schloesing was shot down above the Somme in his Spitfire on 13 February 1943. Badly injured, he made good his escape before being hidden by members of the French Resistance. The Resistance network nursed him to a level of fitness whereby he was capable of escaping back to England by the Comet escape line into Spain and Gibraltar by crossed the Pyrenees. Schloesing is seen in his Spitfire aircraft with the Free French symbol painted on the aircraft's fuselage.

40

Ely became the first service hospital to have a maxillo-facial unit which opened in June 1942. It was staffed by a dental officer who had been specially trained at the emergency medical hospital at East Grinstead. By the time Ely hospital was running at full-strength, it could provide hospital services for over **40** aerodromes from the nearby Bomber Command bases. By the summer of 1943 the overall number of hospital beds at Ely had increased to over **500**. Only patients sent from these hospitals for surgery at East Grinstead had the privilege of joining the Guinea Pig Club.

3

Maxillofacial surgery developed from the dentistry deployed to repair damaged jaws, it became relevant to Polish Sergeant Ludvik Skoczylas. He was a

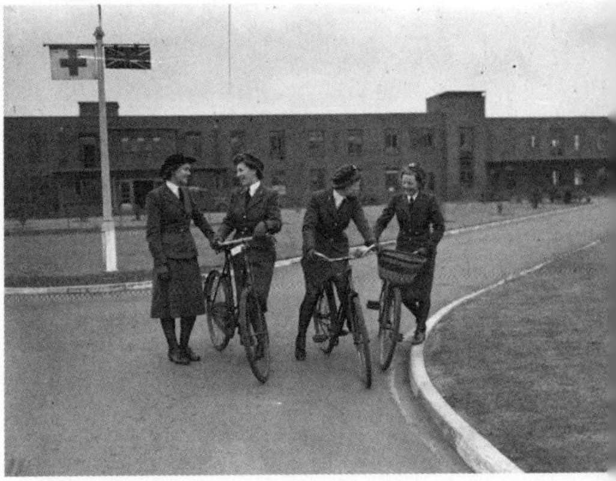

The Royal Air Force Hospital at Ely, opened in 1940 which later provided a burns unit for over **40** operational aerodromes within a **50**-mile radius of Ely. Archibald McIndoe selected many burn patients from this hospital to be treated at the Queen Victoria Hospital. Four off-duty nurses are seen with the extensive hospital behind them.

qualified pilot amongst a group of cyclists on 2 April 1942, pedalling back to their quarters in Bramcote which was a Bomber Command station located in Warwickshire. It was after dark when he was hit by a car, with the collision or subsequent fall fracturing his jaw. Ludvik was initially treated at the Cosford hospital and then transferred to the East Grinstead Hospital on 8 April where the injury required **3** operations to be undertaken. Ludvik is thought to be the first Guinea Pig club member whose admission originated from riding a pedal cycle.

1,130

One air gunner came to grief not in the air but on the ground, in the darkness of the blackouts of 1940. George Harrison was knocked over by a motor car on 17 March 1940. He received a fractured leg, scalp and forehead injuries which needed five operations to repair under the supervision of McIndoe's team. The wartime blackout caused widespread inconvenience, particularly for pedestrians at night. Road accidents increased dramatically with **1,130** deaths occurring in September 1939 alone.[27]

121

In June 1939, all local authorities had received a copy of the Air Raid Precautions Circular number **121**. This circular advised and instructed upon the steps to be taken by local authorities to assist traffic movements and safety during the blackout. These included painting white lines along road centres, marking kerbs, trees and bridges with white paint, screening all illuminated direction signs and pedestrian crossings.

19

The number of Guinea Pigs admitted to the Queen Victoria Hospital as a result of car accidents.

1

Australian airman William J. Cooper was complying with blackout regulations in his bathroom in August 1944 when he slipped, fell and lacerated his right leg. The Leicester Royal Infirmary Hospital transferred him to the Queen Victoria Hospital in September 1944. The necessary surgery took place with **1** operation. He flew as an observer in Transport Command.[28]

2

The second occasion where a pedal cycle was involved and resulted in an admission into the Queen Victoria Hospital involved a Royal Air Force Medical Officer, William Henry Casswell Spooner.[29] He was struck down by a pedal cycle causing facial injuries. The accident occurred at Cheadle, Greater Manchester on 1 August 1941. The accident caused sufficient injuries which resulted in Spooner, meeting Archibald McIndoe at East Grinstead just **2** days after the incident. His facial injuries are ill defined, as are any surgical operations undertaken. However, Spooner was a fellow Licentiate of the Royal College of Physicians. This made him a rather unusual patient. He was no doubt the only member of the Royal College of Physicians to occupy a bed in Ward Three as a patient, making him undoubtedly a unique Guinea Pig.[30]

12 The number of Guinea Pigs who were admitted to the Queen Victoria Hospital with injuries sustained which involved a pedal cycle.[31]

3 The most decorated member of the Guinea Pig Club was Air Marshal Richard Atcherley KBE, CB, CBE, OBE, AFC and bar, also mentioned in despatches **3** times and a recipient of the Norway Cross, instituted by King Haakon VII in 1941.[32]

3 Group Captain Atcherley had most unexpectedly become a Guinea Pig whilst in command of Kenley aerodrome in early 1942. On 26 May, he was flying a Spitfire on a reconnaissance over Dover when a lone Luftwaffe fighter attacked and disabled his aircraft. He escaped by parachute, landing safely in the sea where he was rescued by an air-sea rescue Walrus. Richard Atcherley had sustained a wounded left arm inflicted by the guns of the enemy fighter. The injury was operated upon at East Grinstead where he underwent **3** operations.[33]

8 The second most decorated military ranked member of the Guinea Pig Club was Wing Commander, later Air Vice Marshal Harold Bird-Wilson. He received **8** significant medals during his military service in the RAF, the CBE, DSO, DFC and Bar, AFC and Bar, Dutch DFC and the Czech Medal of Merit. Bird-Wilson had crashed in 1938 and suffered severe facial injuries, including the loss of nose tissue. Those injuries saw him becoming an early Guinea Pig, operated on four times by Archibald McIndoe. The last occasion was in October 1939, making him one of the first Guinea Pigs. However, on 24 September 1940 he was again shot down and parachuted out with burns over the English Channel. He was rescued from the sea and initially admitted to the Royal Naval Hospital, Chatham. There is an ill-defined entry in relation to his readmittance to the Queen Victoria Hospital in 1940.[34] In January 1944, he attended a course at the Command and General Staff School, Leavenworth, in the United States. On returning to the United Kingdom in July 1944, he later

led the Perranporth Spitfire Wing with Fighter Command, flying Mustangs at Bentwaters. He was the youngest Wing Leader to serve in Fighter Command.[35]

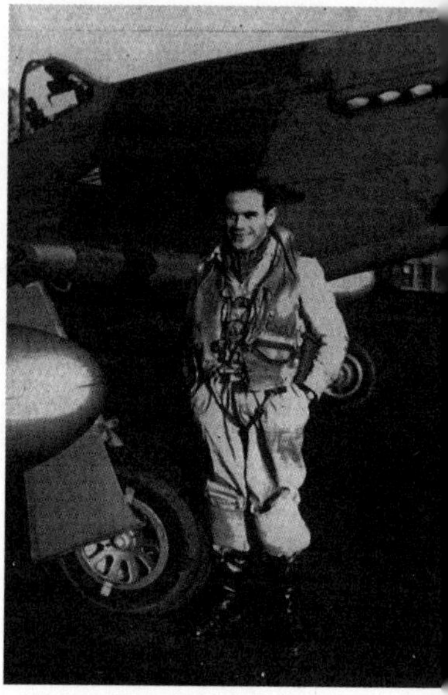

Wing Commander Bird-Wilson standing next to his North American Mustang aircraft at Bentwaters, Suffolk. The fuselage bears the pennant of 'Wing Commander'. Bird-Wilson commenced his operational service fighting in France and during the Battle of Britain.

37

Bird-Wilson was also the Guinea Pig who had the longest period of military service, serving for **37** years between September 1937 to 1974.

18

The third most decorated military rank member of the Guinea Pig Club was Air Commodore, later Air Vice Marshal Cole OBE, DSO, MC, DFC. Adrian Trevor Cole of the Royal Australian Air Force served in the RAF. He sailed with the Royal Navy to act as air adviser to the combined staff controlling the raid upon Dieppe in August 1942. Two enemy fighters attacked his destroyer which was twice bombed. Cole was on the bridge when a shell splinter struck him on the jaw. Another splinter pierced his shoulder blade. Aged 47, he was amongst the oldest serving military individuals to receive surgery for his wounds at East Grinstead. An official history of the raid notes: 'The *Calpe* was attacked by enemy fighters and her bridge was shot up causing several casualties including Air Commodore Cole. "Cole received severe injuries, including a shattered jaw". Initially admitted to Haslar Naval Hospital, he was quickly transferred to the East Grinstead Hospital. "I knew that a broken jaw needed at least four months in hospital,'" Cole later recalled. "This meant that I was sure to lose promised command of a fighter group within Fighter Command which I was to have taken over immediately after Dieppe. Seeing how disappointed I was, Mr. Macindoe [*sic*] said he would see what could be done." McIndoe was true to his word, and in just **18** days, from wound to medical board, Cole was soon pronounced fit for flying duties – "Probably a world record for mending a fractured jaw"'. In October 1942, Cole was appointed Air Officer Commanding, Northern Ireland, with the rank of acting Air Vice-Marshal. He returned to Australia in May 1943. In

January 1945 he assumed the post of the Royal Australian Air Force Liaison Officer on the staff of the Supreme Allied Commander, South East Asia. Cole served in this role until the end of the war. Notably he was Australia's senior representative at the formal surrender by the Japanese in Singapore on 12 September 1945.

1 The pre-war American-born, Canada-resident pilot Paul Yettvart Davoud had flown in the fifteenth annual flying Pageant at Hendon near London in July 1934. On the outbreak of war Paul Davoud began instructing at the Central Flying School in Trenton, Ontario. By early 1941, he had risen to the rank of Squadron Leader and was the Assistant Chief Instructor. Paul Davoud later took charge of a Night Fighter Squadron flying the Bristol Beaufighter in the United Kingdom. Davoud took part in combat operations and in June 1942, he was mentioned in dispatches within the King's Birthday Honours List. He became a Guinea Pig after one of his Beaufighter's engines failed at a critical point when landing on 17 February 1943. The crash resulted in burn injuries to his face and hands. He was admitted initially to Rauceby Hospital, and then transferred to Queen Victoria Hospital on 9 March 1943. He returned to operational flying and survived the war, likely becoming the most highly decorated Canadian Guinea Pig. Group Captain Davoud's decorations were the DSO, OBE, DFC with two mentions in despatches and the Dutch Commander of the Order of Orange Nassau with swords. Guinea Pig Paul Davoud also received the French awards of the Croix de Guerre with Palm Leaf, and the Legion of Honour.[36]

3 On 10 February 1942, **3** occupants of a car at an operational airfield had the misfortune to have an aircraft propellor slice into their vehicle. One occupant was instantly killed whilst the remaining two passengers were significantly injured, one of whom was a Canadian Beaufighter pilot Orvel Dove. He sustained a broken femur, head lacerations and the loss of three fingers. He spent over **3** months in hospital recovering from the injuries before it was decided that he should go to East Grinstead and see a plastic surgeon. The surgeon Ross Tilley operated on him and straightened some displaced facial tissue, removing some of the scarring. Tilley also improved the hand injury to provide greater dexterity. Orvel was a Guinea Pig who returned to flying, but his injuries influenced the medical board to limit his flying within Ferry Command, delivering single-engined aircraft to nominated airfields.[37]

18

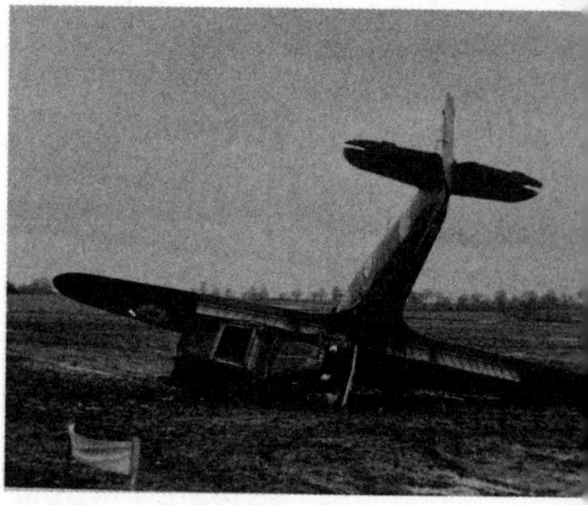

Landing and take-off accidents at aerodromes occurred in many circumstances. This collision involved a Spitfire landing and colliding with a motor car which was upturned in the collision. It is not known if any victims suffered significant injury.

William Towers-Perkins, the founding Guinea Pig Club secretary, was resident in the East Grinstead hospital for over **18** months. Within that time, he was sedated on the operating theatre for ten operations. The burn injuries inflicted upon him on 11 September 1940 prevented his return to operational flying. Towers-Perkins was shot down south of Tunbridge Wells. He parachuted to safety, wounded and burned, and was admitted to the Kent & Sussex Hospital in Tunbridge Wells before becoming a patient of Archibald McIndoe. He was discharged from East Grinstead to the Royal Air Force Hospital at Torquay on 6 May 1942, but was readmitted to East Grinstead on 8 August 1942 for additional treatment to his burn scarring to his face and hands.

3

Aleksander Paszkowski had suffered his injuries at Hemswell airfield on the night of 18 August 1941. His Polish pilot, taking off on an operation to bomb Duisburg in a Wellington bomber prematurely operated the retraction of the landing gear. Insufficient height and gravity forced the aircraft back to earth and the lower fuselage contacted the runway whereby it burst into flames. The bombs on board exploded instantly killing two crew members and injuring others including Paszkowski.[38] It appears he continued to serve and would eventually meet with McIndoe in East Grinstead **3** years after the accident. Archibald McIndoe performed one operation to the healed scarring to his face in January 1945. He was by then identified as a commissioned officer Antoni Paszkowski and became another Polish Guinea Pig Club member.

2

Peter Rathbone ap Ellis crashed in a Tiger Moth training aircraft accident in 1942. Little else is known other than he was hospitalised for **2** years before a new nose was created under the guidance of Archibald McIndoe. At the rank of Wing Commander, Peter ap Ellis retired from service in November 1969.[39]

1

It took just over **1** year between injuries inflicted upon Henry Rutherford Crombie and his admission to the Queen Victoria Hospital. He was injured on 12 August 1941 whilst flying to attack a power station in Germany. His face was struck by Luftwaffe ordnance, probably anti-aircraft flak during the operation. The loss of an eye was immediately obvious to him and his crew of his Blenheim aircraft. His injuries had occurred over Cologne making the return flight traumatic and painful. The facial reconstruction surgery was addressed in seven operations by Archibald McIndoe. Henry Crombie had been admitted to East Grinstead on 12 September 1942. That same day, the King approved the award of the Distinguished Flying Cross to him. He took to wearing a frosted lens in a pair of glasses to alleviate his eyesight disfigurement and he became a celebrated character within the Guinea Pig Club.[40]

332.63

The fastest Guinea Pig to have flow pre-war was Richard Llewellyn Roger Atcherley. He was selected as a member of the Royal Air Force High Speed Flight which was tasked with flying Britain's entries in the 1929 Schneider Trophy Air Races. The race was held over the Solent and the Isle of Wight. Flying Officer Richard Atcherley flew the team's second Supermarine aircraft but was disqualified for crossing inside a pylon at a turn during the race. Flying Officer Henry Waghorn flew the other Supermarine. They broke the world air speed record, flying at a speed of just over **330**mph. Another aspect of the work of the High-Speed Flight also occurred in 1929, when Atcherley took part in the King's Cup Air Race which they won. Atcherley became a Guinea Pig in 1942 and later rose to Air Marshal rank.

1942

Dutton Homestall, the Dewars' country house was a popular place where Guinea Pigs spent time recuperating. They occasionally greeted famous people like Clark Gable, the film star. Gable had volunteered to serve in the American Airforce and visited Dutton Homestall in **1942**. He had graduated as a Second Lieutenant and thereafter made a motion picture of aerial gunners in action as well as flying operational daylight bombing operations.

16

On 7 August 1941, Guinea Pig Timothy Walshe, based on the Isle of Lewis, the largest island of the Western Isles of Scotland, flying Coastal Command Hudson aircraft, collided with an Avro Anson at Stornoway. Both aircraft were on intersecting runways. The Hudson had its tail chopped off and immediately caught fire. Walshe

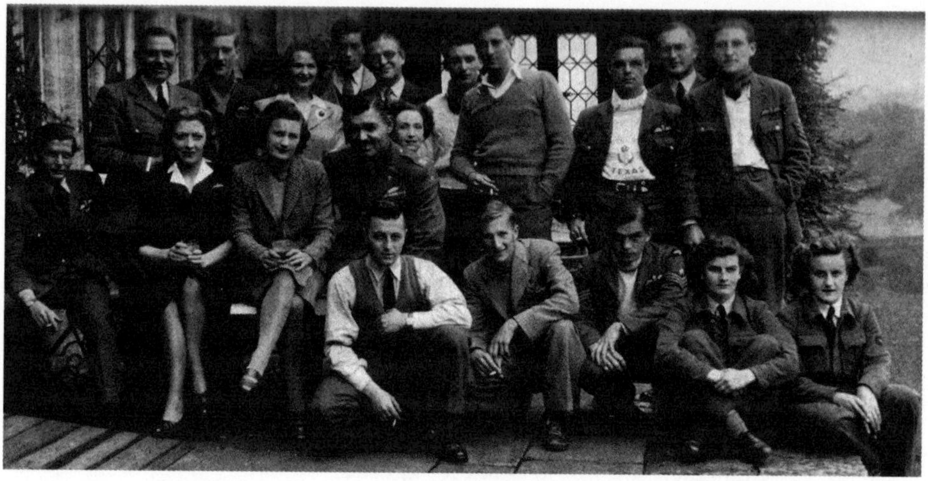

Clark Gable, Hollywood film star, in 1942 at Dutton Homestall. Theatre Sister Jill Mullins is seated second left to Gable, with McIndoe standing behind him.

was knocked unconscious and suffered severe burns before he was pulled from the wreckage. He arrived at East Grinstead in January 1942 for surgery to burns upon his face, scalp, hand and legs. His rescuer from the flames received the George Medal, the recommendation providing details of those events. 'Pilot Officer Alexander John Nicholson was a passenger in an aircraft which was involved in a collision whilst taking off. The aircraft immediately caught fire ... Ammunition and pyrotechnics were exploding and the whole front of the aircraft was in flames but Pilot Officer Nicholson, with complete disregard for his own safety, re-entered the aircraft and making his way forward, found the wireless operator [Tim Walshe] whom he managed to drag to the door when an explosion occurred which blew Pilot Officer Nicholson a distance of twenty yards. The wireless

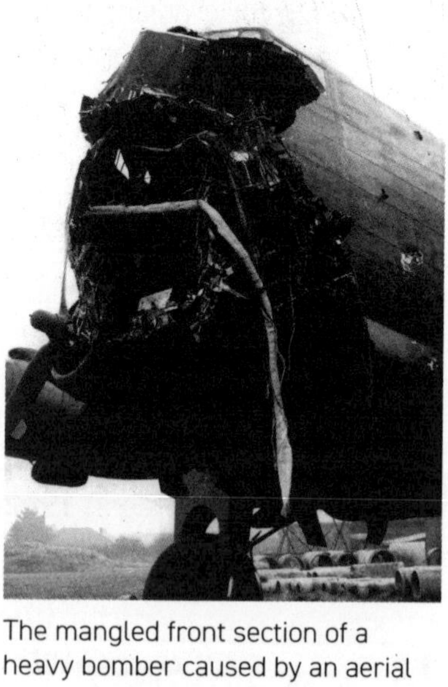

The mangled front section of a heavy bomber caused by an aerial collision. Many Guinea Pigs were operated upon for crush and tear injuries inflicted upon them in collisions and crashes throughout the war.

operator was finally extricated by others but without doubt, his life was saved by Pilot Officer Nicholson's gallantry.'[41] The injuries sustained by Timothy Walshe required **16** operations undertaken at East Grinstead Hospital.

5 Canadian Henry Ernst, a Bomber Command rear gunner, experienced a most unfortunate incident flying over the Devon countryside on 29 January 1943. It occurred whilst completing his **5th** operational mission. His Canadian crew had been on an operation to bomb the submarine pens at Brest, carrying a 4,000lb high explosive bomb. Electrical storms, and heavy icing over the target prevented the release of the bomb. Forced to carry the stuck bomb back in the bomb bay, they crossed the south-west coast of England but unintentionally flew over Plymouth where the anti-aircraft gunners opened fire upon them. The bomb subsequently released itself exploding in the open countryside. The crew decided that Exeter was the best option for safety and the Wellington circled three or four times over where the crew thought the airfield was to be found. Suddenly the aircraft hit a hillside and exploded with four crewmen instantly killed. Henry Ernst and George Beauchamp survived, both badly injured and burnt. Their miraculous escape is undocumented however Henry Ernst was taken to Exeter Hospital where he regained consciousness five days after the crash. He had severe facial burns, a dislocated hip and spinal injuries. He was transferred to the Queen Victoria Hospital on 16 February 1943. By a remarkable set of circumstances, in the adjacent bed next to Henry was his fellow crewmember George Beauchamp who was suffering from third degree burns over his arms and legs.

47 Sergeant Henry Herbert Standen was an observer in the crew of a Hampden light bomber and was about to embark on an operation to drop a sea mine on an enemy waterway target on 14 December 1941. Another Hampden was also to take off, carrying a similar mine at Scampton airfield. A minor collision occurred between the aircraft which was sufficient to create a fire in his aircraft.[42] The ensuing fire resulted in the mine exploding. The explosion wrecked both aircraft, although remarkably nobody lost their life. Henry suffered the worst of any injuries sustained that day. These are best described by a most unusual recommendation for a George Medal, dated 31 March 1942.

'Sergeant H.H. Standen was admitted to R.A.F. Hospital, Rauceby, on the 15th December 1941, following a flying accident at R.A.F.

Station, Scampton, and remained under treatment at Rauceby until the 4th March 1942. He had sustained very severe and extensive burns of face, hands and legs, his hands being burned to the bone. It was necessary later to remove his right eye as a result of the burns sustained. The burns caused four secondary haemorrhages for which blood transfusions were necessary. Sergeant Standen suffered from prolonged and very severe pain which he bore with most exemplary courage and fortitude. The remarkable stoicism and grit which he displayed under such severe physical and mental stress were an inspiration to all medical staff, patients and visitors. His one desire was that he should eventually be fit to resume flying. The medical officers and nursing staff who treated Sergeant Standen unanimously consider that he was the most courageous, long suffering and grateful patient they have ever known. I know from my personal knowledge of this airman, that he would have put up an equally gallant fight in action against the enemy. I strongly recommend therefore, that the outstanding courage and selflessness shown by Sergeant Standen whilst a patient in R.A.F. Hospital, Rauceby, should be recognized by a suitable award. It is considered that the granting of such an award would be a well-deserved consolation and comfort to Sergeant Standen and his parents. I am of the opinion that the morale of all patients, particularly those under treatment for disabilities similar to those sustained by Sergeant Standen, would be materially affected for the better by knowing that the example set by Sergeant Standen had been recognized and rewarded. I consider furthermore, that the granting of such an award to a patient, for bravery whilst in Hospital, would be most favourably received by that large and important section of all classes of the community keenly interested in and sympathetic towards our gallant aircrew patients.'

This recommendation was submitted by the Group Captain, Royal Air Force Hospital, Rauceby on 31 March 1942. No doubt Squadron Leader Fenton Braithwaite had been most instrumental in the submission process. The surgeon's recommendation for a George Medal was undoubtably exceptional and unique. However, the authorities concluded that stoicism was not enough to grant the award. Henry Standen arrived at the Queen Victoria Hospital in April 1942. It commenced a journey of an additional **47** operations for him to endure and he became a significant character within the Guinea Pig Club. Henry Standen's name appeared in the Queen's Birthday Honours list 1982. In recognition of his services as editor of *The Guinea Pig*, he was recognised by being awarded the MBE.[43]

10 One Guinea Pig was recommended for the highest award of gallantry possible, the Victoria Cross: George Frederick Dove, an airman who had already received the Distinguished Flying Medal in 1941 for previous gallantry. The events on the night of 14 February 1943, flying as a mid-upper gunner, saw his Lancaster aircraft flying to Milan in Northern Italy are best described by his Station Commander: 'By his cool, calm and determined valour, Flight Sergeant Dove has added yet another act of heroism to the epic of the Royal Air Force. In spite of flames, which were roaring through the mid-upper turret, he displayed a complete disregard of his own safety in a perilous situation and continued to man his guns with such grim determination, and to handle them with such accuracy, that the enemy fighter burst into flames and undoubtedly was destroyed. Thereafter, he descended from his turret into the flames which must, by now, have seemed to him inextinguishable, to attend to the Rear-Gunner. Despite the fact that to attach his parachute and bale out through the aft door of the fuselage was a simple matter and a ready escape from the raging fire, he deliberately abandoned this chance of saving his own life and proceeded past the door to extricate the Rear-Gunner from his turret. This he did successfully regardless of his own suffering from second degree burns about his face and hands. His object achieved, he rendered valiant assistance to the remainder of the crew in subduing the flames. Thence onwards, Flight Sergeant Dove displayed fortitude of the highest order by making no mention of his injuries to his Captain or crew, so that their attention should not be distracted from their duties, but remained quietly unattended on the rest bed until a safe landing had been completed. I regard Flight Sergeant Dove's indomitable courage, skill and fortitude as exceptional, and one worthy of the award of the Victoria Cross.' His Lancaster had made an emergency landing at Tangmere in Sussex where he received attention in the sick quarters. He was taken to the Queen Victoria Hospital on 17 February 1943,

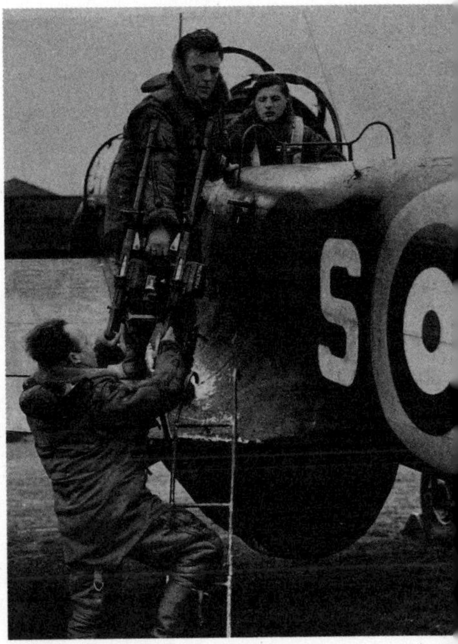

A Hampden crew seen loading the gunner's weapons into his rear-facing turret.

suffering from second-degree burns about his face and hands. Whilst under the surgical care of Archibald McIndoe, the award of his gallantry was communicated to him at East Grinstead. It was published officially in *The London Gazette* on 23 March 1943. George Dove had been recommended for a Victoria Cross but he was to receive a Conspicuous Gallantry Medal (Flying) as directed by the Commander in Chief of Bomber Command. George Dove became one of only **10** men to be awarded the combination of the Conspicuous Gallantry Medal and the Distinguished Flying Medal. Uniquely he is the only Guinea Pig have been recommended for a Victoria Cross.

7

Gerald Figuiere, a French pilot, was a patient at **7** various hospitals who attended to his facial lacerations inflicted by anti-aircraft flak shrapnel when he was shot down over Rouen in France on 26 August 1944. That day Allied aircraft heavily attacked transport targets in France including crossings over the Seine River. Figuiere was treated at a French Military Hospital, a General British Hospital, Dryburn Hospital in Durham, Newcastle General Hospital, Callay Castle Hospital in Northumberland and finally at the Hexham Hospital before eventually being sent to East Grinstead in June 1945. Four operations by Archibald McIndoe were required before he could return to his liberated country. Gerald Figuiere remained a loyal and grateful French Guinea Pig Club member throughout his life.[44]

37

Three men being carried in a Beaufighter aircraft was not a normal occurrence. Operationally, a Beaufighter was crewed by a pilot and navigator sitting in tandem. However, Corporal Frank Gourley

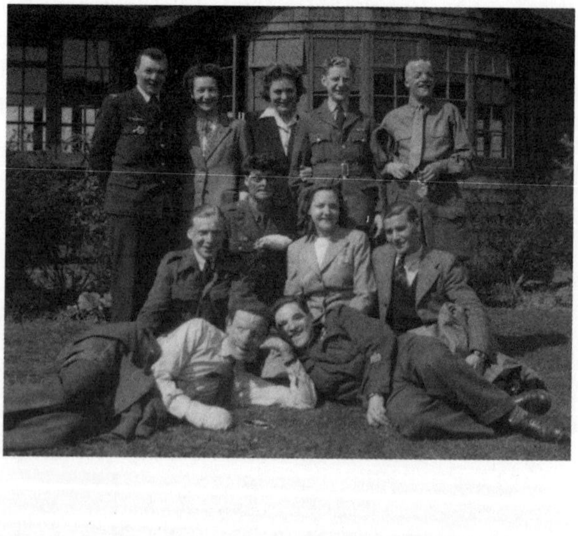

Guinea Pig Sid McQuillan sitting middle left. Standing left, wearing what appears to be a French pilot's uniform, is more than likely the Guinea Pig Gerald Figuiere. Both men were admitted to the hospital within a few months of each other in 1945. Photograph taken showing the 'Maud Barclay Rooms' in the hospital grounds. Maud Barclay was in the League of Friends to the Queen Victoria Hospital.

carrying aircraft inspection documents on a short transit flight joined a Beaufighter crew on 13 December 1943. He squeezed himself into a position behind the navigator. The Beaufighter commenced to take off but it swung sideways and the pilot lost control, with a wing tip striking the ground causing a cartwheel crash. The Beaufighter caught fire and Flight Sergeant A. J. G. Thomas, the pilot, was killed, Flight Lieutenant F. Quinn, the navigator, was injured and Frank Gourley suffered serious burns to his face and hands. Frank Gourlay's injuries became badly infected and five months later in May 1944, Archibald McIndoe brought him to East Grinstead from Rauceby Hospital. Guinea Pig Frank Gourley endured a significant **37** operations undertaken on his burn injuries.[45]

1 William Herbert Mills is the only Guinea Pig to be awarded the Distinguished Flying Cross flying in the post-war Malayan conflict. William had previously experienced a lucky escape on 9 August 1944 when taking off from the temporary airfield at Bognor Regis in Sussex. He was flying the American Mustang fighter when he enthusiastically retracted the undercarriage without enough height, the aircraft's weight saw it dip and crash onto the runway where the Mustang burst into flames. He was extracted but not before receiving burns to his face, arms and back. William was admitted to the Queen Victoria Hospital that same day and naturally became entitled to wear the Guinea Pig badge. He remained in service as a pilot and rose in the ranks. His post-war service in Malaya as a Squadron Leader and his award in 1955 was in recognition of gallant and distinguished service.[46]

7 Canadian Leo Tremblay, flying solo on 26 May 1943 on what was his second night flying training flight, suffered a crash as he attempted to take off. His small Miles Master aircraft burst into flames causing burns to Tremblay's hands and legs. Fellow Canadian surgeon, Ross Tilley at East Grinstead and Archibald McIndoe both applied their surgical skills during his **7** months' residency at the Queen Victoria Hospital. Despite the best care, Leo's right leg had to be amputated at the thigh. He was repatriated to Canada on the hospital ship RMS *Lady Nelson* early in 1944.[47]

3 **3** airmen from the crew of a Halifax heavy bomber simultaneously entered the Queen Victoria Hospital in October 1943. They had been returning home from an attack against Frankfurt Germany. Their aircraft crossed the English coast on two engines and crash-

landed in a field near Biggin Hill and burst into flames. Sergeant Hobbs sustained second degree burns to his face and hands. Flight Lieutenant Warren had similar injuries. Flight Sergeant Edmondston had slight second degree burns of the right cheek and nose. All the casualties were admitted to the Kent and Sussex Hospital shortly after the crash. The uninjured members of the crew returned to their unit on the following day. The three burn victims were transported to the East Grinstead Hospital and admitted together on 5 October. The patients were registered as V. H. R. Hobbs who underwent six medical surgeries for his burns. P. S. Warren who underwent four surgeries and W. S. M. Edmondston whose surgery is unknown. However, this Guinea Pig William Scott Minto Edmondston received the Distinguished Flying Medal acknowledging his completion of **44** operations as an air gunner against some of the enemy's most highly defended targets.[48]

30

Lieutenant Vladimir Razumov became the only Red Army pilot to become a Guinea Pig Club member. The Soviet Air Force 'Voenno-Vozdushnye Sili' experimentally developed their large Tupolev TB-3 long range bomber to carry 'piggy back style', two pilots in their I-16 SBR fighter aircraft. These could be carried significant distances in order to attack distant targets. Captain Vladimir Razumov was selected to fly the TB-3 carrying the fighters mounted upon the upper wings. These pairings were known as the experimental 'parasites' in 1940. Only four TB-3s were modified, and were regarded as the 'Special Mission Squadron SPB' in the Russian Baltic Force. In 1941 the unit operated from the Evpatoria Air Base in the Crimea. The first deployment flown by Razumov was to carry the fighters to attack the Constanza Oil Depot in Romania. This was followed by an attack upon the Romanian Chernovoda Bridge. Flying to Romania and returning to Odessa required an all-round flight of **450** miles.[49] Following close to **30** operations, the parasite flight was discontinued. The TB-3 was subsequently flown to the Caucasus in Southern Russia. At a time unknown, Razumov was shot down flying on the Eastern Front suffering from burns inflicted over Novorossiysk, in Southern Russia, and became a prisoner of war. Major David Livingstone Charters a Royal Army Medical Corps man previously captured in Greece in 1941, undertook as best possible treatment for prisoners of war with burn and eye injuries. He knew of McIndoe and had connections to him through the International Red Cross. Charters came across Razumov and assisted him. In all probability this was the first effective medical treatment he received. Charters provided a basic British uniform for Razumov and facilitated his recovery to Britain amongst the many repatriating patients and prisoners of war. David Charters worked tirelessly in particular treating eye injuries within several prison camps against great adversity.[50] Vladimir eventually arrived at the Queen Victoria Hospital in April 1945, where amongst other treatments, both of his eyelids were reconstructed by Jerry Moore, and thereafter by McIndoe. Razumov received a pedicle graft from his arm to his chin, a rebuilt nose and surgery to the scarring to his face. In July 1946, as his treatment was reaching completion, he had grown accustomed to wearing the uniform of a British Flight Lieutenant and was regarded as a model Guinea Pig patient and was capably learning English. Razumov unexpectedly received a visit from a Soviet official which unsettled him but he disclosed nothing to anyone in the Queen Victoria Hospital. Sometime later, he was visited once more by two Russians from the Soviet Embassy. They went for a walk in the grounds and Razumov never returned to the hospital.[51] Enquiries with the Russian Embassy by Archibald McIndoe were met with negative responses. His disappearance brought great sadness to McIndoe who personally wrote to the Russian address given by Razumov, but never received any replies. Vladimir Razumov had officially flown with the 2nd Special Squadron of the 32nd Fighter Regiment, based on the Crimean Peninsula. He was one of only four pilots who flew the parasite piggy back long-range aircraft. His fate in the hands of the Soviet dictator Stalin in 1946 remains unknown. However, collaboration and treason by Russian prisoners of war was inevitably met with sentences of lengthy forced labour in these times. There is some confusion over the exact spelling of this Russian pilot's name. Vladimir Rasumov is what is shown on the Roll of Honour at East Grinstead.

53856 Christian Boissonas, a French officer serving in the Free French Air Force was aboard a Special Duties Flight Whitley on 25 July 1941.[52] He was a passenger engaged in testing early secret communications equipment. Three French personnel and an Air Ministry official were involved, possibly from Whaddon Hall, the Communications division of SIS (or MI6, as it was more widely known at the time). The Controller was Brigadier Richard Gambier-Parry. One of their best-kept secrets was the use of air-to-ground contact to agents in occupied Europe as well as secret radar using a short-range radio navigation system used for the dropping of airborne forces and supplies. Shortly after taking off, the aircraft suffered engine failure and crashed, with all eight occupants in the aircraft suffering injuries. Boissonas was admitted to the local hospital in Newmarket, then Ely and subsequently into the Queen Victoria Hospital at East Grinstead for treatment to his burns to face and hands. The admittance records importantly recorded his service number **53856** and age of 30. Having recovered from his injuries, Boissonas served in the French 3rd Parachute Chasseur Regiment known in the British Army as the 3rd SAS Regiment, involved in the operations of the Liberation of France and The Netherlands. In August 1944, he was parachuted into France to harass German forces. Eighty-five men of this French unit were dropped into the operational area of Sarlney, Savigny and Messey to link with the local Resistance forces and protect the Allied forces after the American breakout from Normandy. The SAS party destroyed bridges and cut both rail and road links successfully. On 4 September 1944, Boissonas, the only Guinea Pig to serve in the Special Air Service was killed attacking a German convoy. Sixteen men in total from the unit were killed. Capitaine Boissonas was seen running towards the enemy, but he was cut down after a few steps, falling on the edge of the Laives road. His life is commemorated at the SAS War Memorial, Sennecey-le-Grand, France.[53]

1

Czechoslovakian Guinea Pig Alois Siska was posthumously awarded his country's highest military decoration – The Order of the White Lion. He had fled the German invasion of his country in 1939. Whilst in Hungary he was detained but managed to escape and reached Yugoslavia, and then on to Beirut where he enrolled in the French Foreign Legion. This was a common event amongst both Polish and Czechoslovakian escaping airmen volunteering to serve amongst other foreigners as non-legionnaires. Siska eventually reached England where he joined the Free Czech Air Force. All Czechoslovak airmen were enrolled into the Royal Air Force Volunteer Reserve. The official agreement between the Government of the United Kingdom and the Provisional Czechoslovak Government was signed on 25 October 1940. Alois Siska commenced retraining in Wellington twin-engined bombers and also learnt English before flying bombing operations over occupied Europe. His first operational flight was on the night of 10 September 1940, however, during what was to be his final operation to Wilhelmshaven Germany on 28 November 1941, they were struck by anti-aircraft gunfire. Returning home their port engine caught fire making the bomber uncontrollable and the crew ditched into the North Sea. Siska hit his face on the cockpit controls causing injuries but managed to be amongst **5** of the **6** crewmembers who escaped from the aircraft before it sank beneath the waves. It was the height of winter and **2** members of the crew died from exposure in the survival dinghy before the remaining survivors were washed up on the Dutch coast **6** days later. Alois Siska received basic medical treatment for his injuries which by that time included frostbite and gangrene. He was later moved to a German prison camp before being taken to Prague to face charges of high treason and espionage against the Third Reich. The charges related to the German annexation of his country which declared it a 'protectorate' of the Reich. Czech citizens were classified as citizens of the Reich and those Czechoslovaks who fought against the Reich were deemed to be traitors. Charged with high treason and espionage, he was unexpectedly sent to Colditz Castle awaiting court martial and possibly execution. Siska was imprisoned in Colditz for ten months. Following his eventual liberation, he was sent to East Grinstead in June 1945 for treatment for his severe frostbite, receiving treatment over a two-year period. In addition to becoming a Guinea Pig, Alos contacted the Goldfish Club to report that his life had been saved by the rubber dinghy. He was a remarkable survivor and long after the war in 1963, he was called to be a witness at the trial of the Nazi lawyer, Hans Globke in East Berlin. Globke had been instrumental in causing Alois to be charged with treason. Communism induced and imposed tremendous hardship upon Alois Siska, the communists considering him to be tainted with capitalism. Only after the fall of communism in 1989 did he gain his freedom once again. He would proudly discuss being both a Guinea Pig and Goldfish Club member at any opportunity. During his final years, he spent time lecturing schoolchildren on his wartime experiences and regularly attended reunions of the Guinea Pig Club. In 1996 with President Vaclav Havel, the last president of Czechoslovakia, he was introduced to Queen Elizabeth II and the Duke of Edinburgh the then president of the Guinea Pig Club at Prague. He also had

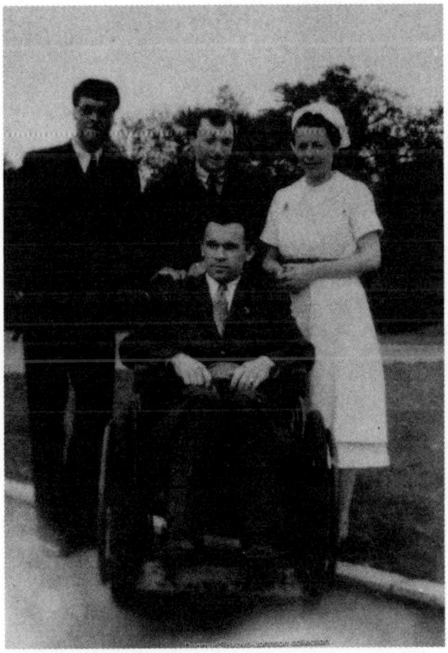

Czechoslovakian Guinea Pig Alois Siska seen in a wheelchair in the grounds at the Queen Victoria Hospital with two other patients and a nurse. (*Free Czechoslovak Air Force Associates Ltd. Dagmar Siskova-Johnson collection*)

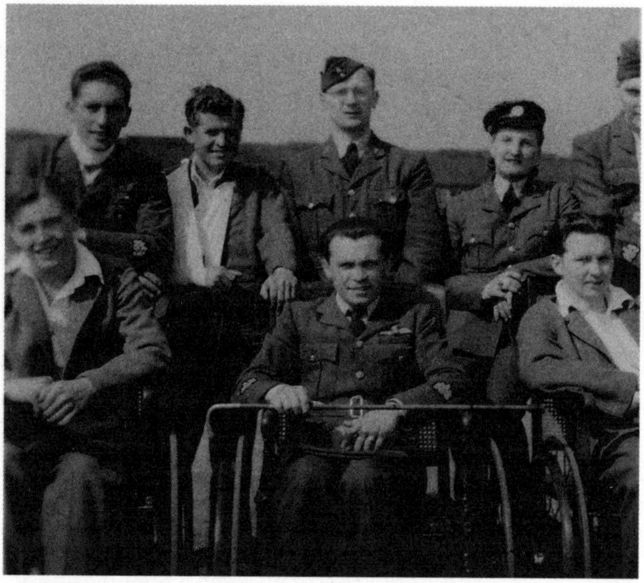

Czechoslovakian Alois Siska, wearing the uniform of a Royal Air Force Warrant Officer with pilots' wings, in company with **2** other wheelchair patients and a mixture of standing patients and medical staff. (*Free Czechoslovak Air Force Associates Ltd. Dagmar Siskova-Johnson collection*)

a street named after him, Generala Sisky in the Modrany District Prague. He died in 2003, an extraordinarily brave and spirited man.

1

The only member of the Guinea Pig Club from the Meteorological Flight service in Coastal Command was Maurice Buttler. On 10 February 1943, his crew broke low cloud off the French coast to find themselves over a convoy of German ships who opened fire upon them. Their aircraft was damaged and set on fire. The pilot managed to crash-land on the French coastline at Camaret Harbour, Brittany. Unfortunately, the additional fuel tank fitted for the endurance of lengthy flights, ruptured and exploded. Maurice was in close proximity to it. The four crew were taken to the naval hospital at Brest. Maurice had suffered severe burns to his face and hands and he was a patient in Brest for a considerable time before being transferred to the Luftwaffe Hospital in Paris. He received treatment for over **6** months and was finally sent for interrogation at the Luftwaffe Dulag intelligence camp in September 1943. Maurice arrived at the Stalag prison camp in Bad Soden in October 1943. His eye injuries appear to have been medically treated in the prison camp by the previously mentioned Royal Army Medical Corps officer, Major David Livingstone Charters. Maurice was medically repatriated to England via Sweden in September 1944 and sent to the Queen Victoria Hospital in East Grinstead on the recommendation of Major

Charters. Maurice underwent seven operations upon his scar tissue and eyelids, qualifying him for his Guinea Pig Club membership.

23

French pilot Robert Bagard endured **23** surgical operations, having had a mid-air accident flying in North Africa on 2 February 1944. The United States Air Force had supplied the French Armee de l'Air with several Bell P-39 Airacobra aircraft for defensive duties over the African ports at that time. It is assumed Bagard may well have been flying such an aircraft, however the records for this French pilot are limited in detail. He arrived at the Queen Victoria Hospital on 16 February 1945. It is known that Capitaine Robert Bagard attended the Guinea Pig Club reunion in 1954.

1

Australian Neil Lambell was flying over occupied Europe when he was struck by shrapnel in the face. The injury required **1** surgical operation which entitled him into membership of the Guinea Pig Club. It also led to him being recommended for the Distinguished Flying Cross, the recommendation read: 'As Air Bomber Pilot Officer Lambell has completed many operational sorties over enemy territory. He has participated in attacks on some of the enemy's most heavily defended targets including eleven sorties against Berlin … On one occasion during an attack on Berlin he was hit on the face by a piece of shrapnel whilst making his bombing run, but, undeterred, he released his bombs at the correct time and it was not until his aircraft landed at base that other crew members of the crew realised he had been injured.' His nose had sustained significant injury. The records advise of his admission into East Grinstead on 9 April 1943.

123

During 1944, **123** men joined the Guinea Pig Club having had their injuries attended to by surgery.[54]

170

In total there were over **170** international Guinea Pigs, making up more than a quarter of the club's total membership.[55]

8

Heavy bomber Flight Engineer Alan Morgan had the unfortunate experience of incurring frostbite on his hands whilst flying over Germany on 20 February 1944. After battle damage, his aircraft's main door blew open and the wireless operator lost consciousness with a problem due to his oxygen supply. Alan removed his gloves to fix the fault, but the external temperature was minus **45** degrees and Alan suffered severe frostbite to his fingers. Frostbite is effectively a burn injury to tissue inflicted by freezing. After his arrival at East

Grinstead on 23 February, McIndoe tried to save as much of his damaged hands as possible. The fingers were beyond recovery, therefore **8** had to be amputated. McIndoe's surgery created stumps which allowed limited movement. Five operations were required and with great will power and determination, Alan returned to operational ground duty as a training officer. He gained employment against adversity and as a Guinea Pig, he delighted in the annual reunions.[56]

2

One Luftwaffe night fighter created **2** Guinea Pigs from within one Stirling heavy bomber crew. On 21 February 1945 the bomber crew anticipated a regular and safe landing having successfully completed their operational flight. Disaster struck from immediately behind and on the aircraft's port side. Raking gunfire came from a Luftwaffe intruder. Both cannon and machine-gun fire from the enemy night fighter penetrated the length of the aircraft. Sid McQuillan, the wireless operator, immediately reported a fire within the aircraft. The emergency escape hatch above the pilot's position was opened whilst Sid McQuillan opened the astrodome emergency exit. Flames and thick fumes were being sucked out of the hatches above the heads of the sheltering men. As the aircraft's landing gear contacted the runway, Sid McQuillan grabbed a fire extinguisher from the cockpit, it was an impulse action but the extinguisher was by then burning hot from the intense heat. He suffered terrible deep burns to his hands. As the fiercely burning Stirling came to rest everyone escaped. Flight Sergeants, McQuillan and Vince had both suffered burns by attempting to use the extinguishers. The front fuselage section of the bomber was dripping molten metal as the cockpit area was totally consumed in the flames. The rescue fire service tackled the fire. Sadly, the body of the rear gunner was found in the remains of the aircraft at the aft section, in all probability killed in the first burst of enemy gunfire. Sid McQuillan and Doug Vince simultaneously joined the Guinea Pig Club with their injuries. Sid McQuillan endured **10** operations overall at East Grinstead, [57] including a pedicle graft from his ear which proved successful.

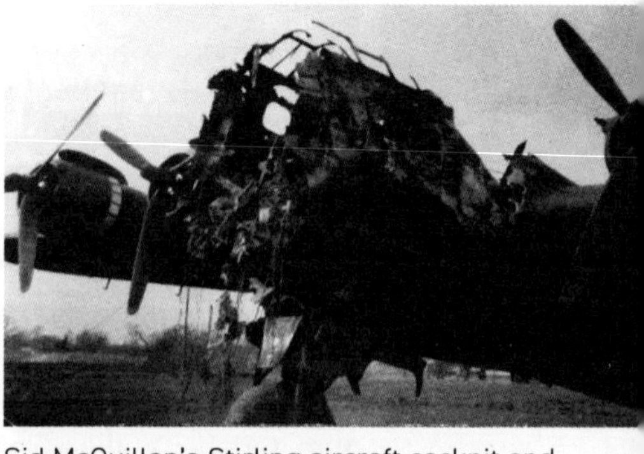

Sid McQuillan's Stirling aircraft cockpit and mid-fuselage area destroyed by fire.

45 The Guinea Pig Club knows of only **3** of its membership who officially became members of the Goldfish Club which recognised the survival of airmen who ditched into the sea. One of these was Sidney McQuillan whose sea ditching occurred on 27 August 1944. His Stirling bombers port inner engine failed and when the propeller parted from the engine shaft and smashed into the adjacent port outer engine some **45** miles from the South Coast of England, an emergency ditching was inevitably going to take place. In the darkness, the heavy bomber struck the water. The impact smashed the Perspex nose and water cascaded into aircraft. The rush of water pushed Sid McQuillan straight out through the broken astrodome and he came to the surface not that far from a dingy that had auto inflated. **5** crew members all joined Sid in the dingy, most having suffered a few minor injuries. Two hours later, a small boat with two occupants was sighted, but despite shouting and waving to the men they were reluctant to approach. Sid then shouted out to them in his Yorkshire accent the names of the entire Aston Villa football team, resulting in the small fishing boat finally approaching their dinghy. The fishermen were from Selsey in Sussex and they set about making efforts to return everyone back to shore. With all eight men aboard the small fishing boat the engine of their small fishing boat stopped working. The oars were then used as the only means of progress. They beached at around eight o'clock in the morning and used the local Post Office telephone to report their situation. Sid McQuillan and this particular crew would never fly together again. The exclusivity of becoming both a Guinea Pig and a Goldfish was never embellished by Mr McQuillan. He was a humble man that the author was proud to have known as a friend for several years.[58]

2 Harry Jenson Morson was the second Guinea Pig who was also a confirmed member of the Goldfish Club. He had been jointly awarded the Distinguished Flying Medal on his fourteenth operation against the enemy. The recommendation stated. 'In November 1940, Sergeant Morson, captain, together with wireless operator, Sergeant Cleverley were in an aircraft which had successfully attacked a target in the vicinity of Berlin. On the return journey, intense anti-aircraft fire was encountered over Hamburg which caused damage to the aircraft, eventually setting the starboard engine on fire. In spite of this, Sergeant Morson set a direct course for base, which necessitated flying across the Heligoland Bight. Although many difficulties were overcome, he was unable to maintain the aircrafts height and was finally forced down into the sea. With

great skill and devotion to duty, Sergeant Cleverley maintained full wireless communication, keeping his base constantly informed of the position. He was undoubtedly responsible for the successful rescue action which was subsequently taken.'[59] Harry Morson then joined the Guinea Pig Club following an engine failure on 22 May 1943.[60] Whilst test flying a Typhoon fighter, he crashed in what was a notoriously heavy aircraft near Dalbeattie town in the county of Kirkcudbrightshire in Dumfries and Galloway, Scotland. He received significant burn injuries which necessitated **4** operations at the East Grinstead hospital. The injuries were sufficiently bad that after his recovery he was discharge from the Royal Air Force in 1944 on medical grounds.

3

The **3rd** known Goldfish Guinea Pig was the irrepressible character who was to feature prominently at every annual meeting of the Guinea Pig Club, Dennis 'Tubby' Taylor. He flew in a Wellington bomber and in late 1941, when returning from his third operation from Germany, his aircraft was shot down off the Dutch coast. The crew ditched into the sea and survived adrift in a dinghy for nine hours before being picked up by the Germans. Dennis Taylor received basic treatment for shrapnel wounds upon his face and thereafter became a prisoner of war for the next three years. He applied for and became a member of the Goldfish Club by having escaped death through the use of an emergency dinghy. In January 1945, Dennis Taylor was among the many thousands of Allied prisoners of war that were forced to march from the prison camps in Poland, westwards into Germany when the Soviet forces pushed the Germans into retreat from the Eastern front. He survived that great hardship and it became an unexpected occurrence to also join the Guinea Pig Club when his facial injuries caused by the shrapnel required the expert attention of Archibald McIndoe following his repatriation from the prison camps. **8** operations reconstructed his face with great

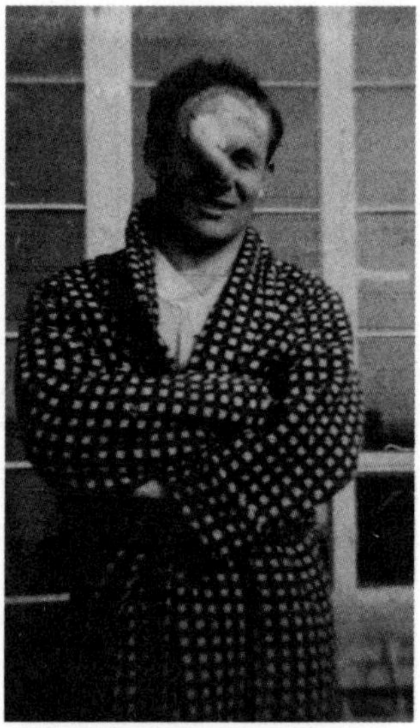

Dennis Taylor, known as 'Tubby' Taylor, with tube pedicle graft after his initial surgery.

success. A tube pedicle procedure resulted in a most successful repair of his disfigured nose. Tubby Taylor was the membership secretary for the Goldfish Club for more than **20** years and he was a staunch supporter of the Guinea Pig Club until his death in 1995.

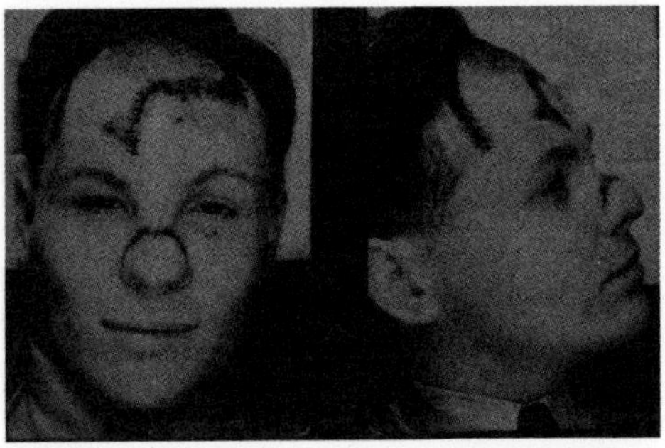

'Tubby' Taylor following surgery after the successful use of his pedicle to rebuild his nose.

14

Canadian Guinea Pig Richard Turnbull spent **14** hours in a rubber dinghy in the company of another survivor from a Wellington bomber which had crashed into the North Sea on 17 January 1942. The crew were attacking the German port of Bremen when an engine fault developed into a fire which induced the untimely and unexpected crash into the sea. The Observer Corps reported an aircraft believed to be a Wellington coming down on fire in the sea close to the coast at Skipton North Yorkshire. In the morning word was received that two of the crew had been picked up by a British destroyer. They were Flight Lieutenant D. R. S. Scrivens and Sergeant R. I. Turnbull of Digby, Nova Scotia. Both were suffering from exposure and frostbite, and Turnbull had a broken nose. These extracts from a letter sent to Wing Commander Fenwick-Wilson from Scrivens provide a personal account of the accident. It was written from Sheppey County Hospital, Kent: '... my hands have thawed enough to let me write, although my feet are still swollen. We are both covered in cuts and Turnbull had his nose straightened to-day and seems quite good. It will probably be a fortnight before we both can walk again, as we were pretty bad when we were picked up ... Well, as to what happened – we crossed the coast and started climbing and about half an hour later Squadron Leader Keddy said the starboard engine was duff. I sent a message to base and thought no more of it. We jettisoned the bombs. Ten minutes later the captain told Masse [the second pilot] to go back and pump oil as we had no oil pressure and told us to get our chutes ready as the coast was ahead of us, and we were at 2,000 feet. Just then the engine caught fire and I went forward and let the second wireless operator out of his turret. He came out and went back, and as I shut the door again I was thrown on the floor and covered with water. After crawling around the bomb hatch for about ten minutes trying to get out, someone fell on top of me and rolled off and I shot straight to the surface. I should think the nose turret fell off completely or something, as I can't imagine I went up through the hatch. On reaching the surface the rear of the kite was still floating and I spotted the dinghy with Turnbull clinging to it. I swam over to it and after several unsuccessful attempts, I found I had my chute harness on, so I got it off. Turnbull was already in the dinghy and with his help, I scrambled in. Our hands were so frozen we couldn't open the rum bottle, the torch didn't work, one distress signal didn't work, and the other we let off when we thought we heard a motorboat, but no good – we froze for fourteen hours before we were picked up. They were very good on the ship. We saw no sign of the others after reaching the dingy.' (A copy of this letter was forwarded with the Squadron Diaries to H.Q. R.C.A.F.[61]) The greatest of fortune came to them when the Royal Navy destroyer sighted their rubber dinghy. On 31 January 1942, Richard Turnbull was admitted to the Queen Victoria Hospital. Archibald McIndoe operated on the injuries he had received, the result of having smashed his face into the cockpit instruments which had displaced his nose. However, the long immersion of his feet in water also caused a medical condition which were rectified by McIndoe. Following his full recovery, the Canadian Guinea Pig Richard Turnbull's subsequent medical board returned him to limited flying service until he was repatriated to Canada.[62]

14 Frederick Holbrook Mahn and Clyde Homer Jay both graduated at Harvard University. Frederick was an American by birth and had emigrated to Canada. Both friends volunteered into the Royal Canadian Air Force in October 1940 and qualified as pilots. Both men were assigned to England in Coastal Command, flying Hampden bombers on anti-shipping patrols. However, Clyde Jay was killed in a flying accident in March 1942 and was buried on Thorney Island in Sussex. Frederick Mahn commenced operational flying in May 1942. On 4 June 1942, Frederick departed North Coates aerodrome to conduct anti-shipping patrols off the Frisian Islands along the Dutch coastline. In poor weather the port engine on his aircraft suddenly failed and they ditched into the sea. Three of the **4** crew survived and were able to reach their small survival dinghy. The details surrounding the crash and ultimate rescue of Frederick Mahn are explained in the following Air Ministry News Service release, dated Saturday 20 June 1942: [63] 'Fourteen days in an open dinghy on the North Sea, the almost unbearable distress of watching two comrades die before his eyes without being able to aid them, the terrible pangs of hunger and thirst – all these were suffered and conquered by a young American member of RCAF 415 Squadron, Pilot Officer Holbrook Mahn, now recovering from his ordeal in hospital.' The story is one of tragedy and great heroism. His rescue finally came **14** days after ditching when the Royal Navy, spotted the dinghy. Frederick Mahn was recovered and taken into hospital where it was discovered in addition to his burnt hands, he had gangrene in both of his feet due to prolonged immersion in sea water. He was taken to the Queen Victoria Hospital at East Grinstead and spent the next **18** months recovering having had both his legs amputated below the knees. Edward George Buller from Coastal Command had the responsibility of researching ditched airmen accounts. He visited Mahn in Ward Three investigating the man reported in the press as eating a seagull to survive adrift in the North Sea. Ironically in June 1943, Edward Buller found himself admitted to the Queen Victoria Hospital. He found himself lying in bed next to Mahn having sustained significant facial injuries in a ditching incident. Frederick, known as 'Hoke', developed a friendship with nurse Betty Marguerite who cared for him in the ward. They later married in the local Church. The wedding party celebrated at the Whitehall rooms.[64] He studied Engineering at Cambridge and the couple had a daughter but on 5 March 1946, he succumbed to an infection that took his life at Addenbrooke's Hospital, Cambridge. His wishes to his wife were for his ashes to be placed with Clyde Jay who had been buried at St Nicholas Church, Thorney Island Sussex. Uniquely, Guinea Pig Frederick 'Holk' Mahn has an inscription at the base of Clyde Jays Commonwealth War Cemetery headstone. Edward Buller is formally recorded as a Guinea Pig on the Roll of Honour board whilst Frederick Mahn is not. The author assumes this error occurred due to his untimely death in 1946.

R62692

No details could be found to confirm previously-published accounts of Canadian pilot Edward William Smith, having become a Goldfish Club member through a ditching incident. Using Smith's service number **R62692** as a unique reference. It was established that on 11 September 1941, his aircraft had crashed at the boundary of Topcliffe airfield whilst practicing pilot dual-instruction, part of a night flying exercise.[65] The approach to land was incorrect and the pilot attempted to climb away too steeply, the aircraft stalled and crashed into the ground. Three of the crew were killed, whilst two were injured. Edward Smith sustained a broken jaw and burn injuries which led to his admission into the Queen Victoria Hospital and membership as a Guinea Pig.[66]

100

Lawrence John Somers from Ontario was a Canadian Spitfire pilot who had accumulated more than **100** flying operations. On 1 June 1942, his Spitfire suffered damage in combat over the English Channel. His aircraft remained airworthy and he was exceptionally fortunate to get home safe. The following day he was on a similar intruder operation. The Luftwaffe fighters intercepted his flight in superior strength and **7** Spitfire pilots failed to return, either plunging into the sea or the pilots parachuting into the waters. Lawrence Somers was amongst them. He went down over the English Channel after his fuel tank had exploded in flames. He escaped by parachute, successfully deploying his rubber dinghy after hitting the water. His burnt hands hindered his ability and his dinghy floated unhindered for two days. A German motor boat located him and he was taken to St Omer hospital for treatment. On 13 October 1942, a prisoner of war post card was received at Lawrence Somers' aerodrome. Lawrence wrote of his recovery in a German hospital. Lawrence was entitled to join both the Goldfish and Caterpillar club. However, no evidence exists to establish if he had made any applications to do so. However, after his repatriation he joined the Guinea Pig Club when he was admitted to the care of the Queen Victoria Hospital in the Canadian Wing on 26 April 1945. He received treatment for his scar tissue injuries upon his eyelids.[67]

0

No details are known in respect of the medical operations provided to Australian Flight Lieutenant, William Mitchell Stanley. He suffered his burn injuries when landing in his blazing aircraft in September 1944. His life was saved by a fellow Australian, Wing Commander Jack Napier Davenport, who was awarded the George Medal for his bravery in the rescue from the burning Beaufighter. Wing Commander Davenport dashed forward, opened the hatch, and struggled to free the pilot who was trapped by his feet. He saved the pilot's life by pulling him out of his flying boots and extracting him from the inferno. The Wing Commander carried him through the flames to safety where he reported upon important enemy convoy shipping movements.[68] The hospital records are vague in detail. However, William Stanley was medically discharged from the Royal Australian Air Force in May 1946.[69] William Stanley is recorded upon the Guinea Pig roll of honour.

7 **7** miles from Dieppe, Canadian Flight Lieutenant Gordon Fredericks faced a dilemma. He had already joined the Guinea Pig Club after crashing in a Hampden bomber in 1941. Having spent months undergoing surgery to his eyes, nose and hands he was fortunate to return to flying duties. On the flight over Dieppe in 1944, his Mosquito sustained damage over Laon-Juvincourt airfield. Gordon received shrapnel wounds to his face and legs, his pilot, Wing Commander Barker, also a Canadian, narrowly avoided a crash into the sea off Dieppe as they escaped the intense gunfire. They glanced the surface of the sea and bounced upwards and at that moment they managed to get a distress call out before the second impact plunged them into the water. Frederick managed to extract himself from the wreckage and also got the pilot free who had been trapped in his seat. Both men managed to climb into an inflated dinghy. They drifted towards the French coast over the course of the night and at seven o'clock the next evening which was 11 May 1944, they signalled two Spitfires overhead of them. The sighting instigated a rescue with the Air Sea Rescue Walrus seaplane valiantly landed close to the French coast and picked up the two Canadians. Fredericks had sustained a broken leg below the knee in the crash. It was an injury usually unlikely to have secured any admission into Archibald McIndoe's care, however, for reasons unknown this Guinea Pig returned to the Queen Victoria hospital once more.[70] The twice-admitted Canadian Guinea Pig Gordon Fredericks undertook recuperation and convalescence after his second series of operations. Archibald McIndoe and his team strongly advocated gainful and rewarding work and for Gordon, his recouperation was undertaken at Reid and Sigrist's, the electrical and aeronautical engineers at New Malden.[71] McIndoe was aware of Gordons Frederick's engineering interest and he also appears to have influenced the opportunity for him to study at Cambridge University. Gordon later wrote to McIndoe reporting his achievement of having attained a 'University First'. This endorsed the appetite that Archibald McIndoe possessed in helping his Guinea Pigs build better lives for themselves.[72] Gordon Fredericks was indeed a most fortunate survivor and achiever in his life.

12 Some Belgian Spitfire pilots flew from England over their home country. One pilot, Jacques Carlier in company within a flight of **12** Spitfires experienced an unexpected intrusion into his flightpath by a Polish pilot, Stefan Kalarus flying a Lysander on Anti-Aircraft calibration duties on 8 January 1942.[73] Jacques Carlier's collision in the air was unavoidable, it occurred over Wales at Plas Gors

Rhosneigr, near the aerodrome of Valley. The Lysander crashed near the golf links at Trewan Sands and was consumed by fire. Jacques had saved his own life by managing a force landing near Anglesey in Wales. His facial fractures saw him admitted under the care of Archibald McIndoe for many months. This Belgium Guinea Pig Club never flew a Spitfire again. However, he was later awarded an Air Force Cross in September 1945 having flown in the Communication Squadron on a special flight, he had been employed on the evacuation of casualties from North West Europe. This Guinea Pig was also awarded the Belgian Croix de Guerre.

16

A metal hook was fitted to the lower right arm of Guinea Pig Ronald Pretty. It replaced his hand which was lost in a Halifax heavy bomber crash during training on 5 December 1942. The Halifax had taken off from Riccall in Yorkshire for a cross-country navigational exercise. Eye witnesses reported that the aircraft was flying low near Scunthorpe. It was observed to bank and as it was getting steeper the aircraft eventually fell to the ground, crashing amongst buildings. The aircraft crashed through the roof of a factory and exploded killing all but one of the crew members. Sergeant Ronald Pretty was critically injured. His face, arm and remaining hand eventually recovered from burns to regain normal use after **16** medical operations. The amputation of his right hand never dampened his spirit. He became a prolific attendee at the Guinea Pig Club reunions. The entertainer and supporter of the club, Max Bygraves at an annual reunion announced his intention to sing his new song called 'You Need Hands'. Ronald's false hand suddenly came skidding across the floor towards the entertainer with rapturous applause.[74] Guinea Pig humour was never lacking at the reunions. Max Bygraves released the popular song in 1958.

327

Bomber Command suffered **327** deaths and the loss of **70** aircraft on 17 December 1943. It was a day when a large force of Lancasters and Mosquitoes had taken part in a bombing raid on Berlin. Returning aircraft from the operation saw thick fog blanketing the country. One air gunner, Warrant Officer James Benbow witnessed his crews Lancaster running desperately low of fuel. They had been diverted to the airfield at Graveley which had a fog dispersal system designed to disperse the cloud and fog using flaming petrol. Pipes carrying thousands of gallons of petrol had been installed down all sides of the runway. The pipes were pierced with holes, from which a fine jet of petrol spurted and ignited. The heat dispersed

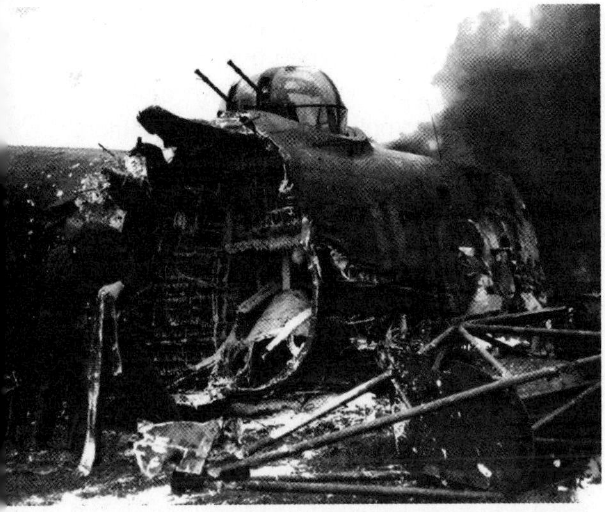

During a training flight in March 1945, this Lancaster heavy bomber suffered an engine failure. The pilot was unable to trim the aircraft to stop the aircraft turning in flight. It landed but swung off the runway, crashing and burning. The fuselage has split apart exposing the central section which has been doused with foam used to quell the flames. Two of the crew suffered injuries. A great number of airmen in training were killed or badly burnt in scenes like this throughout the war.

the fog and cloud, and the glow of the flames provided a flarepath. Unfortunately, due to the conditions on that night there were a number of fatal crashes at and around Graveley. James Benbow's crew crashed at Graveley and their bomber burst into flames. He was the only survivor from that crew. Both of his legs were broken and he had sustained significant burn injuries. James was initially treated at the hospital in Ely before an admittance into the Queen Victoria Hospital where he remained for **14** months. The injuries were of such significance that he was invalided out of the Royal Air Force in early 1945.

12

The number of crewmen who normally manned the large Short Sunderland flying boats which flew from Castle Archdale on Lough Erne, in Fermanagh, Northern Ireland was **12**. On 12 August 1944, one Canadian crew carrying George Willoughby Allen and Martin Alexander Platsko experienced an extraordinary crash after an engine failure. The unit's operational record book explains the events. 'Flight Lieutenant Devine and crew who had just taken off on an operational trip at noon, crashed twenty minutes after take-off at Belleek, County Donegal, Eire … they contacted flying control that oil pressure was high on starboard outer engine and requested permission to jettison Depth Charges in Lough area. The D.C.'s were however jettisoned over land but apparently aircraft could not maintain height on three engines as the outer engine had seized. The second pilot advised that a crash landing was being made. The landing area selected was probably the best in the vicinity being a reasonably level and boggy area. The aircraft struck a small knoll almost immediately on touch down and turned over breaking in two. The aircraft burst into flames and the entire forward section including most of mainplanes burnt completely beyond recognition.' The injuries sustained by George Allen and Martin Platsko resulted in both Canadians being transferred from Halton for burn treatment surgery at the Queen Victoria Hospital thereby joining the Guinea Pig Club. Martin Platsko was repatriated in September 1945 and George Allen appears to have been repatriated home on 27 November 1944.[75]

25th

Archibald McIndoe always donned his operating gown on 25 December in order to carve the Christmas turkey for his patients.

26

Greek-born Stephen Molivadas witnessed the invasion of his country to German forces in April 1941. He escaped to Egypt where the Hellenic air force was reorganised in Cairo. Three Hellenic squadrons were created which joined the Allied air forces. Molivadas became a flying instructor at the Royal Air Force navigation school in South Africa. Later he flew operationally eventually joining the 13th Hellenic Squadron in Italy. From May to November 1944, the activities of the Greek squadrons continued in Italy where bombing, offensive reconnaissance and patrolling missions of strategic importance were carried out. Stephen Molivadas was shot down on 25 July 1944 in Sarajevo, Yugoslavia and taken as a prisoner of war. His burn injuries received little medical care and in March 1945, he was transferred into the custody of the German forces. German troops had evacuated Greece, Serbia, Albania, and Bosnia-Herzegovina during the autumn of 1944. However, German and Croat troops continued to fight in north-western Yugoslavia until the end of April 1945. Stephen Molivades was amongst prisoners freed by Allied troops having been taken to Austria's capital city of Vienna. His injuries were assessed and he was transported to England for treatment. Stephen Molivadas is the only Greek airman to have been treated at East Grinstead. He endured **26** operations.[76] Impressively during his treatment and recouperation in Sussex, Molivadas undertook a post-graduate degree in electrical engineering with the University College London. He was a remarkable member of the Guinea Pig Club.

16

There were **16** Polish Guinea Pig Club members. Jan Adamczyk, Joseph Biel, Franciszek Bielawski, Jerzy Glebocki, Edward Gwardiak, Waclaw Korwel, Zdzislaw Krasnodebski, Antoni Paszkowski, Tadeusz

Podbereski, Alojzy Ratajczak, Jan Stangryciuk, Michal Bobitko, Walenty Heine, Eugeniusz Orchel, Ludvik Skoczylas and M. Szafranski.

0 Polish pilot Witold Jozef Krupa is not officially recorded as a Guinea Pig. He is however quoted as having been treated at East Grinstead Hospital.[77] In Witold Krupa's book, *Flight Through the Storm*: 'On 22 September 1944, Senior Sergeant Pilot Witold Krupa from the 306th Fighter Squadron "Toruński" was involved in an accident. Piloting a Mustang III UZ-E (HB871), he had taken part in air cover for Operation Market Garden the previous day. After returning from Holland, he landed with the squadron at Friston [near Eastbourne in Sussex] and was due to fly back to Brenzett Field Airfield the following day. He crashed the plane during take-off, suffering burns. The pilot was taken to the Princess Alice Hospital in Eastbourne, from where he was then transferred to the Queen Victoria Hospital.' The 306 Squadron records confirm in AIR 27/1674/17 that P784381 Krupa did suffer this accident and his hospital admission is documented. No explanation can be found as to why he is absent from the records as a member of the Guinea Pig Club.

3 James Russell had an explosive bullet round penetrate a hand when flying from Malta in July 1943. Insufficient detail exists to identify any additional information other than after initial hospital treatment, his injury subsequently resulted in **3** operations at East Grinstead. His hand was saved, thereafter becoming another grateful Guinea Pig.[78]

4 At least **4** Guinea Pigs arrived at the Queen Victoria Hospital as victims of high-tension power line flying incidents. The 1st being a Sergeant Dash of which little is known. The 2nd, Aubrey John Hawksworth received the skill of McIndoe in saving the thumb digit on his right hand. Unfortunately, his other portion of hand was lost completely. He developed his art skills and dexterity to become an accomplished cartoonist.[79] The 3rd Guinea Pig was medical student Eugeniusz Orchel from Poland. He escaped Poland and in May 1941 he ventured into unoccupied Southern France, before crossing the Pyrenees and into Spain. From there he sailed to Great Britain where he volunteered to fly in the Royal Air Force and trained as a navigator. During a training flight on 30 November 1942, his Wellington crashed at Monks Kirby in north-eastern Warwickshire having struck high tension power lines. He was thrown clear of the

wreck unconscious and seriously injured. He was only found later that evening and assumed dead. He was taken to the mortuary of a nearby cottage hospital. A Polish Air Force colleague Aleksander Bielecki of 300 Polish Squadron, came to pay his last respects and noticed that Orchel was still alive. Immediate care took place. He had a fractured skull and later developed gangrene in his right hand which required the removal of three fingers. He was taken to East Grinstead where McIndoe undertook additional surgery. With McIndoe's support, Eugeniusz Orchel graduated from the Polish School of Medicine in Edinburgh in 1947. He was granted British citizenship and thereafter worked as a family doctor in Middlesborough.[80] The 4th Guinea Pig was a Canadian air gunner Leslie Caddel. His Wellington bomber struck power lines on 19 July 1942 killing the rest of his crew in the crash. He suffered burn injuries which were operated upon by Ross Tilley, addressing eye, ear nose and jaw issues.[81]

1

Australian pilot, Kenneth John Trask flew the powerful American Mustang fighter aircraft which would lead to his admission into the Queen Victoria Hospital. He came to grief on 13 August 1943 with a fractured jaw and lacerations to his face elbow and knee. The Hospital details disclose his service number as **409347**. Flying Officer Kenneth John Trask, during the summer of 1943 was serving at various airfields including Dunsfold, Weston Zoyland, Woodchurch and finally in October 1943 at Redhill. The squadron records advise he went missing over Cherbourg when his flight was forced to climb through cloud owing to a low ceiling height. Trask lost contact with his flying partnering aircraft and failed to return home, thereby being posted as missing. He lost his life flying Mustang AG547 near Le Havre, France on 11 November 1943, barely three months since having become a Guinea Pig at the Queen Victoria Hospital.

1

Raymond Fowler, Flight Engineer in a Halifax on 24 May 1944 was faced with a challenging engine fire after take-off. A second engine then faltered inducing a crash landing into a field. The crew of **7** all sustained various injuries but for Raymond Fowler burns to his hands resulted in his admission into the care of Archibald McIndoe. His **6** crew who had suffered minor injuries soon returned to operations. Within a short time period, **5** of them would fail to return home from operations. Ultimately, becoming a Guinea Pig for Raymond Fowler may well have saved his life.

1,203

Prisoner of war exchanges were conducted between Germany and Britain from 1943 to late 1944. These exchanges of prisoners, predominantly with debilitating injuries many of which would have been survivors from within Bomber Command. The accumulation of statistics for heavy bomber crew losses within Lancaster, Stirling and Halifax crews commenced in January 1943. These statistics revealed that between January to June 1943, **6,498** men from Bomber Command had failed to return from operational duties. The Red Cross prisoner of war notifications communicated through Switzerland were no doubt responsible for establishing that there were just **1,203** survivors. Statistics are not available to identify how many of those men were repatriated with burn injuries.[82] Undoubtably, amongst them there will have been many who underwent plastic surgery.

8

Official German prisoner of war identification records exist for **8** prisoners of war who became Guinea Pigs. These eight prisoners of war combined required **31** separate operations at East Grinstead Hospital after repatriation to England.[83] They were J. Atkinson shot down 27 June 1944, W. Ball shot down 23 August 1943, J. Biel shot down 8 August 1941, N. Brooks shot down 13 October 1944, M. Buttler shot down February 1943, F. Falkiner shot down 27 October 1941, P. Fitzgerald shot down 5 January 1945 and N. Hallifax shot down 15 May 1940.[84] Four of the above were repatriated before the end of the war. The remaining **4**, Biel, Brooks, Falkiner and Fitzgerald, all remained prisoners of war until liberated from their camps in 1945 by Allied forces.

1

Only **1** person from a crew of **4** survived an accident on 15 April 1943 when training in a Wellington Bomber. It was taking off when a burst tyre slewed the aircraft across the runway into the aerodrome's windsock and the aircraft burst into flames. The survivor from the flames was an Australian Sergeant, Cecil Rhodes. He sustained burns to his face, hands and scalp. Within **5** days of the accident, Cecil was admitted to the hospital at East Grinstead. **8** operations were undertaken and the medical interventions continued in Australia after his repatriation. Sadly, on 21 May 1946, Cecil Rhodes died following what was ultimately his final operation. His details of membership as an Australian Guinea Pig are celebrated on the club's roll of honour at the Queen Victoria Hospital.

3

Only **3** men survived from a Lancaster crew which crashed returning to their base. Canadian Jacob Redekopp became a Guinea Pig as a result of rescuing a fellow Canadian from the crashed bomber on 20 May 1944. They had just completed their 16th successful operation before the crash landing. Jacob was still conscious after the crash and he was able to remove both Owen Jones and Jim Philips from the burning aircraft. As a result of going back inside the burning plane to affect the rescues, he was severely burned. He was treated at Halton before his move to the Queen Victoria Hospital on 15 July 1944. Owen Jones had already arrived at East Grinstead on 26 June. Jacob remained in the hospital for one year before being sent back home to Canada for rehabilitation. Owen Jones received surgery for lacerations to his head, a shattered jaw and burns. Jaw patients inevitably had frames around their beds from which hung weights. Their locked jaws were attached through pulleys to weights which held the shattered jaws under tension. The patients were in a fixed position sitting up in bed which allowed the liquid food to be fed by tubes.

1

Stanley Reynolds and George Fawcett served together flying Beaufighters before converting to the Mosquito aircraft. During operations on 9 July 1944, their aircraft suffered an engine fire which was successfully extinguished. Returning on **1** engine resulted in the landing speed being too excessive. Unsurprisingly, they overshot the runway by some distance lurching through a field and into a ditch. The ensuing crash saw the pilot Reynolds receive lacerations across his face. His navigator suffered a smashed jaw. The aircraft caught fire but George Fawcett's left foot was trapped before he could get free. Eventually both men crawled away as the fuel tank exploded. Dr Tilley and Archibald McIndoe repaired the jaws and rebuilt the faces of this Canadian pair of casualties. Stanley Reynolds returned to flying duty on 11 August 1944 and was finally repatriated at the end of the year. George Fawcett's broken jaw took longer to repair, his repatriation to Canada is unknown.

123

Believed to be the number who became Guinea Pigs in 1944.[85]

24

In February 1944, a clinical conference was held at Hill End, St Albans where it discussed the appropriate use of penicillin in war injuries, and **24** surgeons were present. This conference was the beginning of what eventually became the British Association of Plastic Surgeons.

529

As of 24 July 1945 this was the number of members of the Guinea Pig Club.[86]

31

One outstandingly brave rear gunner was Ronald Vivian. He flew **31** operational missions in 1941, and engaged enemy night fighters on at least two occasions. Eventually a crash landing took place in France where he escaped and managed to reach Spain, returning to England by Gibraltar. Ronald was awarded the Distinguished Flying medal for his bravery. However, in the blackout, whilst alighting from a taxi in December 1944, he lacerated his eyelid, an injury sustained in far less dangerous situations than he had endured flying against the enemy. Archibald McIndoe repaired his injury and he became a Guinea Pig in March 1945.

32

The highest number of facial fractures repaired on one Guinea Pig relates to the Canadian, Lionel Hastings. His injuries were sustained in a flying accident in an Anson aircraft on 15 October 1944. Engine failure and telephone lines induced the accident with him sustaining **32** facial fractures, **3** spinal fractures and both leg and arm fractures. He was regarded as a mashed patient at East Grinstead. He was encased in a body plaster cast and traction kept him bedbound for some significant time.[87]

30

William Foxley was anesthetised **30** times for medical operations undertaken to reconstruct him from injuries sustained on 17 March 1944. Foxley's bomber crashed in flames during a training mission. Foxley managed to escape relatively unscathed but was severely injured when he went back into the burning remains and rescued the wireless operator who was trapped. The plane blew up, killing **3** of Foxley's crewmates. This bravery appears to be unrecognised by any award. His reconstructed face included a glass eye, which glinted when it caught the light. He appeared as a badly burned pilot in the film *Battle of Britain* made in 1969. Bill Foxley was by many, considered to have been the most badly burned airman to survive the Second World War. He added to his medical operation total in January 1949 when his appendix was removed at the East Grinstead Hospital. He had married Catherine Arkell a nurse at the hospital two years previously in June 1947.

1

It appears that Jimmy Buckee was the only member of the Guinea Pig Club who joined directly from having been in the cockpit of a Miles Martinet target towing aircraft. He crashed, receiving burns on

17 May 1944. During his **9** operations undertaken at East Grinstead he formed a lasting friendship with Sister Mary Meally whom he later married in 1951.[88]

6 Uniquely, a crew of **6** survivors from one crashed heavy bomber all joined the Guinea Pig Club together. On 5 July 1944, this crew were dropping supply containers and arms at an area close to the Swiss frontier. On board was Australian Flying Officer Stannus with Flight Sergeants White, Bacon, Marjoram and Smith with Pilot Officers Watkins and Holmes. Having reached the dropping site in bright moonlight, their Stirling was struck by anti-aircraft fire and seriously damaged. In 2016 Harold Stannus provided the author with the details of what took place in their aircraft. 'With one engine out and the second on the same side disabled, the Pilot was forced to fly in a crablike attitude. I advised the pilot to feather the disabled engine to prevent drag. We flew that way for some time and then the load was jettisoned in the English Channel. I had opened the canopy hatch above the pilot while still in flight and let it loose so the opening was free in case we ditched. The aircraft was damaged by flak, the tanks were holed and fire broke out in the port wing root, Flight Sergeant Smith displaying great present of mind, chopped through the fuselage with an axe, thus enabling him to reach the flames with extinguishers, thereby putting out the fire. He then assisted the Flight Engineer in an attempt to repair the damage sustained to throttle and pitch linkages. The Flight Engineer subsequently became overcome by petrol fumes. Flight Sergeant Smith not only carried out his duties as Wireless Operator, but also those of the Flight Engineer and gave frequent petrol and engine checks. Throughout the whole of the trip, Flight Sergeant Smith remained calm and extremely helpful and played a large part in getting the aircraft back to this country. He had advised that all of the fuel tanks were registering as empty and that a ditching was highly probable.' Despite the odds, the crew managed to reach Thorney Island aerodrome on the South Coast of England where they crash-landed. Harold Stannus recalls further. 'The Wireless Operator contacted Thorney Island which was closed and dark for an emergency landing. The base lit their runway lights. As the landing gear was not working, the Pilot aimed for the grass and successfully landed missing concrete pylons and structures in that area but unfortunately the plane skidded across the runway and this created sparks and ignited the fuel. The open escape hatch created a flue for the flames which rushed forward toward the cockpit. The Pilot climbed out first but was sideways and his hips got stuck so I had to help him turn sideways to get out. I then followed the drop from the top of the plane to ground was about 8–10 feet. The navigator lost his life in the ensuing fire whilst the remaining crew all escaped with burns.' Harold Stannus sustained burns to his left hand, left cheek, nose, mouth, chin and neck. Thomas Smith had suffered significant burns to his hands, no doubt inflicted as he fought the initial fire. His recommendation for the award of a Distinguished Flying Medal appeared in *The London Gazette* on 10 January 1945. The recommendation read: 'As a wireless operator this NCO has completed a total of 47 operations ... On one special operation, the aircraft in which he was flying was severely damaged by light flak, resulting in a large amount of petrol entering the fuselage. Flight Sergeant Smith immediately stood by to start the distress procedure as the captain considered it necessary and continued to do so until the aircraft reached the English Coast. The Flight Engineer became affected by the petrol fumes, turning on petrol tanks that had already been emptied and was quite incapable of keeping his log or intelligently watching his instruments. Flight Sergeant Smith manipulated the fuel cocks correctly and watched the engineer's panel in addition to his own duties. The aircraft landed wheels up and caught fire ... After some time in hospital, he re-joined the Squadron with his enthusiasm for operations undaunted in any way.' The **6** crew members who survived all suffered burns of varying intensity. They received initial medical treatment at the nearest local hospital, St Richards in Chichester. The following day they were taken to the Queen Victoria Hospital in East Grinstead. Thomas Smith, Harold Stannus, Douglas Bacon,

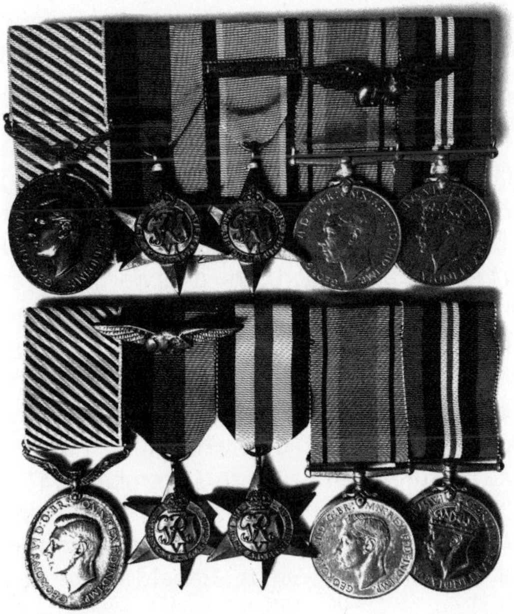

Thomas Smith's medal group together with Frank Webster's medal group. A pair of gallant Guinea Pig Club recipients of the Distinguished Flying Medal. Both awards were for service flying in Bomber Command as a wireless operator and an air gunner respectively.

Charles Watkins, William Holmes and Charles Marjoram all became Guinea Pigs. The remaining member of this crew, Flight Sergeant White became a casualty to the flames and lost his life inside the rear of the aircraft.

2

Hurricane pilot Patrick Wells is amongst the few Guinea Pigs who survived **2** emergency parachute escapes after aerial combat in 1940. It was the second occasion when he sustained burn injuries having been shot down by the famous Luftwaffe fighter pilot Adolf Galland. The award of the Distinguished Service Order for Patrick Wells in 1944 explains his gallantry. 'Squadron Leader Wells has now completed his third tour of operational duty. His first tour was completed during the Battle of Britain, when he destroyed at least two enemy aircraft and was shot down twice. In May 1941, during the battle of Malta, he was wounded for the third time, but after a short period returned to operations, taking part in offensive sweeps over Sicily and low flying attacks on mechanical transport and shipping. Throughout the whole of the Eighth Army advance from El Alamein, he was engaged in patrols over the enemy lines and operations against searchlights and mechanical transport. His courage and devotion to duty have been unfailing in the face of numerous difficulties and setbacks.' After the war, Patrick subsequently lived in South Africa.

8

The number of Canadian nursing sisters who worked the medical wards attending to Guinea Pig patients. They were Matron Margaret Kains and Sisters Marion Patterson, Margaret Peacock, Marjorie Jackson, Enid Faulkner, Curley Vernon, Mons Stapleford and 'Midge' Phillips.[89]

3

3 members of a Whitley bomber crew all became Guinea Pigs on the same day. On 16 October 1941, the crew of **5** were undertaking a night training flight and are believed to have been in the circuit over Croft aerodrome Durham when their starboard engine failed at low height. Their port engine also failed soon afterwards and at an estimated height of only 300ft, the pilot attempted to force-land the aircraft in a field. They crashed and the aircraft caught fire. The crew escaped but three men sustained serious burns, Bertram Owen-Smith, Ronald Frederick Whitehorn and Canadian Joseph Gerard Oliver Dufort. After initial treatment at Rauceby Hospital all **3** men arrived at East Grinstead in late November, early December 1941.[90]

44

The combined number of operations that took place upon the Guinea Pig Club trio of Bertram Owen-Smith, Ronald Whitehorn and Joseph Dufort.[91]

1 Bertram Owen-Smith was inspired by Archibald McIndoe to become a medical surgeon whilst undergoing treatment for his own burn injuries. For nearly two years as a patient, he studied and educated himself to matriculate in medicine. McIndoe supported his ambition to become a plastic surgeon. Bertram made the unique transition from patient to doctor studying medicine at King's College, then Westminster Hospital and later trained with McIndoe for three years at East Grinstead. In 1957, he emigrated to Salisbury, Rhodesia where he practised medical surgery. Bertram Owen-Smith achieved a second unique achievement as a Guinea Pig. In 1964, he stood for election for the Rhodesian Parliament and was elected as a Member of Parliament. He served as one of Prime Minister Ian Smith's backbenchers. He was a remarkable man who died on 6 June 2008, aged 86.[92]

1943 During the war, Leeds Castle in Maidstone, Kent had been providing general military hospital accommodation. In **1943**, the castle extended an invitation to provide respite specifically for Guinea Pig patients as guests of Lady Baillie.

2 Polish airman Alojzy Ratajczak endured **2** flying accidents, both caused by weather conditions. The first incident on 2 January 1943, occurred when the build-up of ice to the wings of his Wellington bomber caused them to crash near Nottingham. Alojzy Ratajczak was treated by Archibald McIndoe and naturally joined the Guinea Pig Club but his injuries remain unknown. His second accident was influenced by an electrical storm over France on 27 July 1945. This incident killed the entire crew when their aircraft flew into high mountains near Lyon.

1 Polish Sergeant pilot Edward Gwardiak became a Guinea Pig whilst flying a Lysander target towing aircraft. Posted to the Isle of Man, he flew the Lysander for air gunnery students. During an afternoon flight on 26 March 1943, accompanied by the winch operator who sat behind him facing rearwards, poor weather unexpectedly reduced visibility. Flying low to view the ground he clipped an obstruction near Gretch Farm, Laxey, causing the aircraft to crash. The injured pilot and operator were pulled from the wreckage by soldiers stationed nearby. Seriously injured and unconscious, Gwardiak was taken to hospital in Douglas and then on to East Grinstead. Injuries sustained included fractures to his arm, skull and face.

Once recovered he was posted to undertake instructor duties at the Polish Elementary Flying Training School in Hucknall.

1

Polish pilot Tadeusz Podbereski was a flying instructor who became a member of the Guinea Pig Club with injuries which are ill-defined in any records. He was the only Polish volunteer to become a Guinea Pig whilst flying a small Miles Master, a British two-seat monoplane advanced trainer. On 19 September 1942, his student pilot was flying the Miles when it hit a tree and crashed on to the White House Farm, in the village of Colston Bassett, near Nottingham. The pilot, Leading Aircraftsman Rewers died in the crash, Tadeusz Podbereski survived and found himself at East Grinstead, becoming one of the few Polish Guinea Pigs.[93]

2

Only **2** men are known to have succeeded in flying again after losing both legs. Douglas Bader was one, but he was not a member of the Guinea Pig Club. The second was Colin Gerald Shaw Hodgkinson who had been accepted for pilot training in the Fleet Air Arm in 1938. He was grievously injured in a flying accident whilst training in May 1939. He had crashed when his Tiger Moth aircraft was struck by another during training. His aircraft fell to the ground at Gravesend in Kent, killing the instructor. Colin awoke in hospital to find that his right leg had been amputated at the thigh, whilst his remaining left leg was severely injured. His face was also damaged, and he had trouble with the sight in one eye. In the weeks that followed, Colin's left leg refused to heal. Coolly and calculatingly, he made his decision and requested that it be amputated.[94] Colin developed a burning determination to prove himself capable of becoming a fighter pilot and flying Spitfires, using Douglas Bader as his example. He was fitted with a pair of tin legs at Roehampton Hospital with the authority's intention for him to be invalided out of service. Leonard Mosley's biography of Archibald McIndoe[95] discloses that Hodgkinson was convalescing at Dutton Homestall when he met McIndoe. The surgery at Roehampton had left unsightly scaring around his left eye. Moreover, once in his care, McIndoe could fight his case to not be invalided out of service. McIndoe engaged with his medical welfare and the Royal Navy. In November 1940, Archibald McIndoe succeeded in getting Hodgkinson reinstated in service. This was primarily where Archibald McIndoe had challenged and instigated the removal of the 90-day rule for military medical discharges. Colin Hodgkinson then joined the RAF and by March 1943 he was capably flying once more. He quickly proved himself as a fighter pilot, until his war ended by becoming a German prisoner of war, another similarity with Douglas Bader. Colin Hodgkinson was captured on 24 November 1943, after his aircraft suffered oxygen failure during a high-altitude weather reconnaissance sortie. He was rescued from his burning Spitfire on the ground in Northern France by two farm workers, losing an artificial leg in the process. After some **10** months as a prisoner of war, Colin was repatriated in 1944 having been deemed by the Luftwaffe as unfit for further duty. Surviving records indicate that he arrived back in Britain on 16 September 1944 and was admitted to the East Grinstead Hospital exactly a month later on 16 October. In total, Colin underwent four operations for the scar tissue lacerations upon his face and a previously unknown fractured jaw. He was an extraordinary member of the Guinea Pig Club.

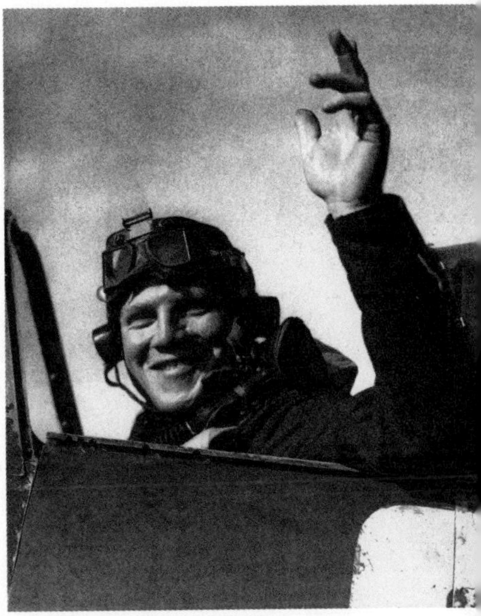

Colin Hodgkinson pictured in the cockpit of a Supermarine Spitfire at an Operational Training Unit on 7 October 1942.

18

Sam Gallop was a pilot who lost the best part of both of his legs in a flying accident. He became a resident Guinea Pig Club in Ward Three for **18** months after an aerial collision whilst flying an Oxford in inclement weather on 9 April 1943. His aircraft fell and hit the ground and burst into flames. By good fortune, he was dragged from the flames which saved his life. He was burnt, his left hand had lost a finger, his jaw was smashed as were both lower legs. His unconscious state would remain for seven days. Both legs needed to be amputated, and for **18** months, there were successive operations. He never flew again but his continued support for all disabled individuals over many years led to him being awarded a Commander of the British Empire in the Queen's Birthday Honour's list in 2002 for services to People with Disabilities.[96]

2

A pair of flying incidents resulted in **2** independent admissions into the East Grinstead Hospital for the previously mentioned Frantisek Truhlar from Czechoslovak. His first accident occurred flying in a Wellington bomber which crashed close to Bentley

Priory, near Stanmore in 1940. Frantisek was admitted to the Queen Victoria Hospital severely burned and frostbitten. Remarkably he later qualified as a Spitfire pilot. He flew operationally once again but on 11 June 1944 returning from France on his **60th** operational flight, he was forced to put his aircraft down near Portsmouth short of fuel. The Spitfire struck an obstacle as it slewed across the ground and burst into flames. Once again he was subjected to burn injuries. Archibald McIndoe welcomed the popular Truhlar back to Ward Three at East Grinstead for the second time.

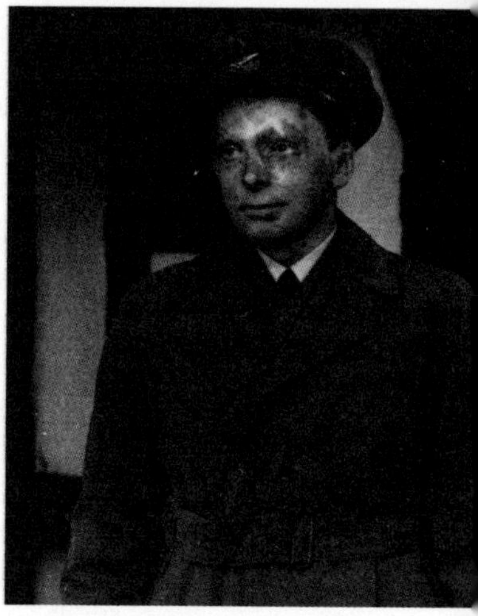
Frantisek Truhlar. His facial scarring is clearly evident in this image.

1 Frantisek Truhlar is the only Guinea Pig to have been operated upon having sustained burns as an Air Gunner in a bomber crew and later as a fighter pilot flying Spitfires.

1 Sergeant Frank Webster appears to be the only Mid Upper Air Gunner flying in Bomber Command who became a Guinea Pig after a fire took hold in the aircraft fuselage directly underneath his elevated position. Despite his burn injuries he beat the fire out with his clothing. The recommendation for the award of a Distinguished Flying Medal to him for his bravery was published in *The London Gazette* on 5 December 1944.

3 One Guinea Pig Club member suffered **3** flying incidents resulting in **3** independent admissions into the East Grinstead Hospital. He was Geoffrey Page, a founder member of the club, first shot down and burned over the English Channel in the Battle of Britain. When flying over Normandy after D-Day in 1944, he collected another nasty shrapnel wound which saw him admitted to the care of McIndoe for the second time. His third injury was at Arnhem. A fractured maxillary antrum in his face saw him back at the East Grinstead hospital. Historically, these three battle periods are amongst the most significant of the Second World War. Geoffrey Page had **17** medical operations and received recognition of his flying bravery by the multiple awards of the Distinguished Service Order, Officer of the Order of the British Empire and the Distinguished Flying Cross and Bar.[97]

1 Shrapnel had the potential to create deep penetrating wounds anywhere on the body. Metal shards originated from many types of weapons during explosions in the air. Service personnel and airmen frequently had the misfortune to be struck by these burning white hot sharp metal fragments which were of various configurations and dimensions. The East Grinstead Museum data upon the Guinea Pigs disclose John Thompson, a soldier serving in Egypt in 1943, is registered as a Guinea Pig having been injured by shrapnel.

5 At least this many Guinea Pigs wrote their memoirs. The first of the wartime memoirs was published anonymously, the author being identified only as 'A Battle of Britain Casualty'. The author was Group Captain Thomas Percy Gleave. Guinea Pigs Geoffrey Page, Jo Capka, Richard Hillary and William Simpson all published memoirs. Richard Hillary's title, *The Last Enemy*, was written after being shot down over the English Channel and rescued by the lifeboat *Lord Southborough* from the Margate boat station on 3 September 1940. Hillary's book met with much acclaim including Archibald McIndoe who recognised the intellect of the author. After pushing many boundaries and rejecting medical guidance, Hillary was later assessed as fit to fly and was posted to an Operational Training Unit at Charterhall in Berwickshire in the Scottish Borders, despite Archibald McIndoe expressing his opinion in writing that Hillary was not ready to resume flying. His Blenheim crashed on the night of 8 January 1943. Both he and his observer, Sergeant Kenneth Fison, aged **38** were killed. Hillary was just **23** years old. Richard Hillary of Trinity College is remembered by an annual literature prize, and a lecture given at his university in his honour.

2 The number of wartime autobiographies penned by one author, William Simpson. The Guinea Pig Club's first newsletter makes mention of a book written by Squadron Leader Simpson, *The Way of Recovery*, a personal account of his own recovery as a Guinea Pig which was published in 1944. Later published was the title One of Our Pilots is Safe.

2 Staff Sergeants Edward Bronski and Edward McGovan were amongst the crew of an American B-17 Flying Fortress which flew to France on 31 August 1943. Two B-17s collided and exploded near the French target whilst other bombers suffered significant damage from enemy defences. The pilot of Edward Bronski's aircraft, Jess Rogers made a successful bombing run over their target. His aircraft sustained damage by debris from an aircraft collision above them as well as flak shortly afterwards. Limping home at a reduced height, shortly before reaching the English coastline, the pilot gave his crew an opportunity to parachute out before more height was lost. Three crewmen jumped from the stricken aircraft before it lost further height and crashed onto the land of Wooten Farm, Polegate, near Eastbourne Sussex. Only **2** men survived the crash, Edward Bronski and Edward McGovan. Both had suffered burns to their faces and hands. Edward Bronski had suffered a leg injury **14** days previously, inflicted by Luftwaffe fighter attacks over another target. The two American airmen were taken to the Princess Mary Hospital in Eastbourne but almost immediately taken to the Queen Victoria Hospital, East Grinstead. These Americans would have stood apart from the predominantly British patients, many of whom would have been very interested in the Flying Fortress bombers flown by the United States Army Air Forces. The **3** crew who parachuted from the aircraft all lost their lives, presumed to have drowned. Staff Sergeants Edward Bronski and Edward McGovan are the only known pair of American airmen who joined the Guinea Pig Club. Additionally, according to a newspaper report, Edward Bronski and Edward McGovan are reputably the first patients operated upon by Archibald McIndoe in the first completed operating room within the hospital's American Wing building.[98]

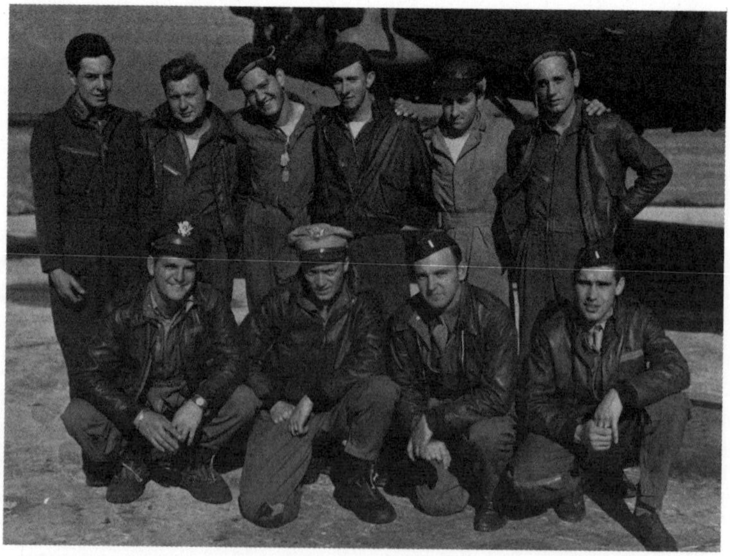

Crew photograph with Edward McGovan standing second left. (*Daniel Bon*)

2 Australian Guinea Pig Warrant Officer Charles Kenneth Gilkes suffered face and hand burns when he was shot down. He was flying his Stirling bomber returning after a sortie over occupied Europe on 7 September 1943. Freeman Strickland, also an Australian who flew Spitfires suffered similar injuries when another aircraft crashed into him as he prepared to take off at Sicily in September 1943. Both Royal Australian Air Force airmen received reconstructive surgery at the Queen Victoria Hospital in September 1944. A year after their respective injuries both airmen were authorised for repatriation to Australia. The **2** airmen are known to have become an inseparable pair of Australian Guinea Pigs.

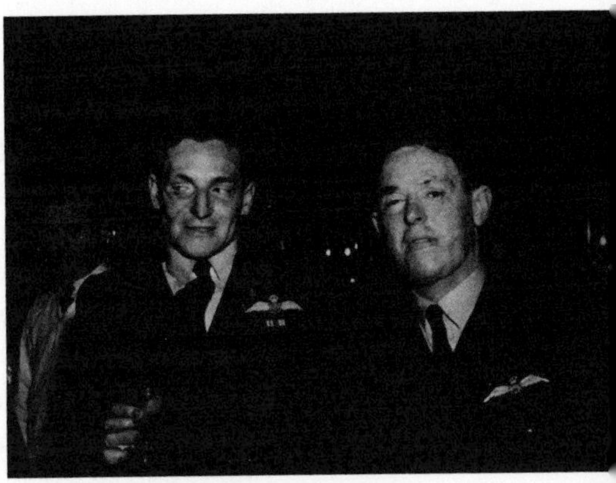

Two Australian Guinea Pigs, Flight Sergeant Charles Kenneth Gilkes and Warrant Officer Freeman Strickland, pictured together in the United States in 1944. This photograph was taken in New York on the home journey. (*Australian War Memorial; AWM2016.767.6*)

1 Eric de Lyon, a Dutch Spitfire pilot under training in the RAF, was the only Guinea Pig accused of treason Erich Henry Johann de Lyon was born on 12 February 1916 in The Hague to his unmarried half-German mother and full German father, Erich Muller. His mother later married the Indian civil servant J. de Lyon and Eric took his family name. Together, the family left to live in the Dutch East Indies. Eric spent his youth in Sumatra and Java, later commencing his military service where he trained as a student pilot. In 1936 he crashed a training aircraft in negligent circumstances which saw him dismissed. Following the German invasion of the Netherlands, the Dutch East Indies districts saw the detention of all German aliens. Eric's German ancestry became problematic. However. he was not detained and was allowed to rejoin his military pilot training which he completed at the end of 1940. Eric de Lyon and Sergeant pilot Harry Kelder also of Dutch nationality were sent to Britain in 1941 to train as fighter pilots in the Royal Air Force. The intention thereafter was to fly in the European theatre of conflict against the occupying German forces. During training, Pilot Officer Eric de Lyon suffered a facial injury on 17 October 1941. He was admitted to the East Grinstead hospital on 21 October 1941, and

the medical intervention he received enrolled him into becoming the 2nd Dutch member of the Guinea Pig Club. The records state the injuries were caused by a blow to the face. The declaration of war by the Japanese in attacking Pearl Harbor on 7 December 1941 induced orders for the three Dutch pilots, Eric de Lyon, Harry Kelder and William John Burk to sail to the Dutch East Indies. During the journey, an order from Vice Admiral Helfrich of the Royal Netherlands Navy diverted the ship to Colombo in Ceylon. The **3** pilots were to be jointly assigned to 18 Squadron of the Royal Netherlands East Indies Army. General Major L.H. Van Oyen ordered the pilots return to the Dutch Sergeant Pilot status. They were assigned to a joint Dutch and Australian bomber squadron under Royal Australian Air Force operational command. In the most vague circumstances during the autumn of 1942, the three Dutch pilots were arrested in Canberra in Australia on suspicion of 'Attempted sabotage, aiding the Japanese and desertion'. By order of the Dutch Military High Command in Melbourne, these pilots were transferred by ship to Colombo to be tried by a specially established Naval Court Martial. The trial took place on board a requisitioned passenger ship that was anchored in the bay of Colombo. The alleged circumstances were so serious, the Naval Court Martial fiscal sought the death penalty or life imprisonment. Much evidence originated from one friend of the pilot William Burk, a friend who reputedly acted as 'agent provocateur' with consent of a supervising officer, the objective of which may well have been to set examples to restore or maintain discipline. The Court President considered the evidence of all charges to be sufficiently present. He did so simply upon the basis of written signed statements carrying convincing evidence. The court's verdicts were – life sentence for the Pilot William John Burck and **20** years imprisonment each for the two sergeant pilots, Eric de Lyon and Henri Kelder. All **3** men were dishonourably discharged from military service. During the years of detention between 10 November 1942 and 30 April 1950, Eric de Lyon and the other two pilots were held in various prisons as war criminals and considered dangerous to the state. Their long-overdue pardons in 1950 saw their release from the Special Prison in Leeuwarden in the Netherlands.[99] After his release, Eric de Lyon was able to get a job as an agricultural pilot flying a light aircraft crop spraying. On 15 June 1976, he suffered an untimely accidental death.

2 Leading Aircraftsman[100] Ronald William Ensor Humphryes was accidentally shot in the right eye with a signal flare gun in January 1942. Signal pistols were mounted on a bracket fixed to the fuselage of aircraft. The pistols fired coloured flares, either when in distress or for identification purposes. The facts concerning the discharge of the flare remain unknown. It must be assumed to have been an accidental discharge. Ronald had **2** operations in 1943 to reconstruct his face and right eye socket. After the war, Ronald Humphryes moved to Hastings in Sussex and became Secretary of the charity Blesma, which provided limbless veterans support for life. In addition, he was also the editor of the RAF newsletter for the Hastings district and a strong supporter of the Guinea Pig Club. Ronald Humphryes is another example of a Guinea Pig who did not meet the requirement of the club rules in that he was not a pilot or aircrew.[101]

1 Flight Lieutenant James Hooper had the misfortune to suffer the loss of an eye when flying his Avro Anson aircraft on 1 September 1943. A bird strike penetrated the windscreen and struck him in the face. The injuries to the eye were such that it was impossible to be saved. He was admitted from the sick quarters at Portreath airfield into the Queen Victoria Hospital on 14 October 1943.

3 The number of operations performed on an armourer, Leading Aircraftsman Roy Francis Haslam, at the Queen Victoria Hospital. Haslam had been serving in Rhodesia on a practice bombing range. In early 1944, a bomb exploded causing injuries on his left side, face and arm and hand. He was attended to at hospitals in Rhodesia, South Africa, Liverpool and Banstead before admission into East Grinstead, becoming a McIndoe Guinea Pig. It is possible that his service in Rhodesia has been interpreted as making him a Rhodesian National within the East Grinstead Museum database. The admission into Archibald McIndoe's care took place on 22 July 1944. Roy Haslam eventually lost his left arm. It appears that this amputation occurred after extensive measures were taken to save the limb which had been injured **5** months previously.

1 The only RAF clerk or administrator to have the honour of being a Guinea Pig was Leading Aircraftsman Norman Hill who was injured during an enemy aerial bombing raid in the Middle East in 1943. He was repatriated and underwent **3** surgical operations by Archibald McIndoe.

1

The only RAF Balloon Operator to become a Guinea Pig was Frederick Ballentyne who was serving at Abbey Wood in south-east London. On 12 January 1941, a bombing raid set an ammunition magazine near their position on fire. An explosion injured Sergeant Ballentyne and two others. Ballentyne was admitted to the Queen Victoria Hospital with what were described as incendiary burns. The first fatality in Balloon Command had been Aircraftsman Philip Hopwood who was killed by a lightning strike. His electrocution by the tethering balloons steel cable was just prior to the Declaration of War. He was therefore denied a Commonwealth War Graves Commission headstone.

1

The Commander-in-Chief of the Polish forces, General Wladyslaw Sikorski, visited the Queen Victoria Hospital on 5 October 1940. Sikorski decorated his pilot Major Zdzislaw Krasnodebski with the prestigious Silver Cross of the Virtuti Militari. This was for his gallantry in flying before fire engulfed his cockpit and his escape by parachute on 6 September 1940. His face and hands carried raw burns as he lay in bed and the medal was pinned to his chest by General Sikorski. The Luftwaffe had previously shot Krasnodebski down over Poland during the invasion of his country in September 1939.

17

The number of individual operations that took place to reconstruct and repair Guinea Pig John Brian Birks. He had previously endured the danger of completing a tour of operations across occupied Europe for which he had been rewarded with the Distinguished Flying Cross. Being rested from operations, he was instructing at an operational training unit in the summer of 1943, when his student pilot accidently collided with an obstruction whilst taxiing. When inspecting the aircraft for any damage a propellor struck him causing significant injuries on 25 July 1943. Three days later, John Birks was admitted to the care of Archibald McIndoe.[102]

2,154

The Avro Lancaster had three self-sealing tanks fitted in each wing, each tank reducing in size from the fuselage towards the furthest small tank at wing end. The total capacity of fuel was **2,154** gallons which was apparently coloured green for identification purposes.

1

One member of the Guinea Pig Club is known to have sustained face, shoulder and arm injuries following the explosion of a stationary Hurricane's fuel tank. Serviceman Graham Lawson is recorded as of South African nationality with a service number 914554.[103] However, this number was allocated to the Royal Air Force and issued in September 1939 at Uxbridge. The injury occurred in June 1941 and Lawson was hospitalised in Gibraltar and later Halton before arriving at East Grinstead in November 1941. He endured **2** operations. His nationality remains definitively unknown.[104]

1 One Guinea Pig member joined the club after the fuel tank in a motor car exploded which occurred in July 1944. Derick Marygold's rank was Corporal, with a ground trade of electrician. Archibald McIndoe accepted Derick into his care **6** months after his injuries. He had previously been treated at Kettering hospital and then Ely where undoubtably he was seen by McIndoe in January 1945. Derick Marygold received **10** operations to repair his burn injuries.

32 Full thickness third-degree burns were inflicted upon the face and hands of American pilot Ward Morehouse Bowyer. These had occurred on 3 November 1943 after his Wellington bomber had sustained damage when training for night landing. An engine failure presented problems in a landing. On the approach Ward Bowyer overshot in the darkness, the aircraft swung sideways and crashed on Loxley Hill, bursting into flames on hitting the ground not far from Wellesbourne airfield. He escaped from the wreckage but returned to rescue a crew member and was severely burnt. Sergeant L. E. Hance was extracted from the crash but died of his injuries the following day. Ward Bowyer's burns on his hands and face necessitated **32** operations by Archibald McIndoe over the following **5** years, He was a volunteer American in the Royal Air Force who originated from Savannah Georgia. After becoming a Guinea Pig and during his recouperation between surgery, he had a number of short stories published. He spent time researching at the British Museum and worked as a reader and writer for the European Story Department of the Twentieth-Century Fox Film Corporation. In addition, he enthusiastically became a prominent supporter and assistant editor of the Guinea Pig Club newsletter. He unexpectedly died at Downing College in 1949 of causes unrelated to the terrible burns inflicted **6** years previously. He had been in pursuance of a literary career and was studying at the college under Dr Leavis. Archibald McIndoe had sponsored and recommended Ward Bowyer's attributes to the prestigious college within the University of Cambridge.[105]

12

Ian Quilter was an observer navigator in the Royal Navy Fleet Air Arm. He had joined 811 Squadron flying anti-submarine patrols protecting Atlantic convoys. Flying from Northern Ireland on 14 of July 1944, the engine failed on his Swordfish aircraft during take-off at Limavady. The aircraft crashed and immediately burst into flames. He suffered significant burns to his hands and face. Taken to Cosford, the Royal Air Force hospital in Birmingham for treatment, Archibald McIndoe invited him to be admitted to the Queen Victoria Hospital at East Grinstead. **12** operations were performed upon his injuries. Ian Quilter was one of only **2** naval aviators to become a Guinea Pig.[106]

11

An unusual combination of crew and passengers consisting of **11** Polish military personnel were on board a Wellington bomber on 11 July 1942. The aircraft was authorised to visit the operational training unit at Bramcote in Nottinghamshire. Pilot Officer Mazurkiewicz was the pilot and his cousin, Lieutenant Pietraszak of the Polish army was amongst the passengers. After a successful visit, the contingent departed from Bramcote but as they did so, the aircraft suffered an engine failure. This resulted in a crash with the aircraft bursting into flames. The pilot, his cousin and Sergeant Kostorkiewicz were killed whilst the other Polish servicemen Franczak, Ziolkowski, Peski, Wodzinski, Jaruszewski, Szpek and Jan Adamczyk were injured, the latter sustaining facial and hand injuries. A delayed admission into the Queen Victoria Hospital resulted in Jan Adamczyk being admitted in August 1945. Among his injuries, it transpired he had sustained a broken neck. This Polish Guinea Pig became a naturalised British citizen after the war and his recognised name thereafter was John Adam. He was a stalwart member of the Guinea Pig Club until his death.[107]

1

Squadron Leader Roy Lane was the only Guinea Pig club member to be executed by the Imperial Japanese military forces. This Hurricane fighter pilot had flown operationally from Tangmere airfield in the summer of 1940. The Battle of Britain was being fought with intensity over the south of England and flying his Hurricane, Roy Lane claimed a Luftwaffe bomber destroyed on 8 August. He later engaged the masses of Luftwaffe bombers and fighters over Portsmouth on 26 August when his aircraft suffered critical damage. His Hurricane was on fire and diving to earth upside down. Roy Lane was hanging by his harness straps as he tried to avoided many of the flames. Unable to release himself, he struggled to escape and unable to do so, his fate appeared set as the Hurricane hurtled downwards on fire. Inexplicable events saw him suddenly freed from the cockpit. He assumed the flames had burnt through his harness and he was falling towards the ground. Reaching for his parachute, another horror was exposed. It was no longer where it should have been. With a burnt hand he managed to find the ripcord and deployed the parachute. Roy Lane was hanging upside down with the parachute suspended above him whilst the straps entangled his ankles. He landed on the ground by using his shoulder to take the impact, protecting his head as best possible. His right trouser leg was burnt away and his face was burnt, but to a lesser extent than his right hand which was missing a lot of skin burnt away by the flames. Roy Lane was admitted to the West Sussex Hospital, Chichester and then went to the Queen Victoria Hospital, East Grinstead, where he underwent surgery by Archie McIndoe and became one of the club's founding members.[108] Two years later, Roy Lane returned to fly Hurricanes in the unusual duty of flying from converted catapult contraptions from merchant steamships. Later in 1943, he volunteered to fly in Burma. He had volunteered to operate with the Chindits, as the air liaison officer to Brigadier Bernard Fergusson. The Chindits were operating in Japanese occupied territory but required aerial spotting support. They built an airstrip and provided a Hurricane for Squadron Leader Lane's use. During one duty flight between the forward airstrip and Imphal he was worryingly forced to land near a village **20** miles east of the Chindwin River, the result of a glycol leak. Knowing the danger, he was intent on reaching British lines. He set out through the inhospitable terrain but was captured by the Japanese soldiers and executed on or around 26 April 1944.[109]

24 Sergeant Franciszek Bielawski, a Polish pilot of the Night Fighter Squadron 'Lwowski' flew in the wooden built Mosquito aircraft. On 21 September 1944, together with his British radio observer Gilbert Fowler, he took off from Church Fenton on a training flight. As a result of an engine failure the Mosquito hit a tree, crashed and burned. Both crewmen survived but Bielawski suffered severe burns. He was taken to York Military Hospital, and then Rauceby until he was transferred to East Grinstead, arriving on 5 November 1946. Seven operations were to be undertaken on his neck and body areas. This Polish pilot had a most significant delay of **24** months between his accident and receiving the specialist surgery necessary, thereby becoming a member of the Guinea Pig Club.

2

Jack Calder, one of the Guinea Pig Club's committee members, of 1944 was another man who experienced **2** emergency parachute descents. The first occurred in 1941 when he parachuted into a bog and was interned in Eire for some considerable time. His second misfortune occurred in August 1943, when he sustained significant injuries after his aircraft crashed into the top of a mountain in the north of England. He was taken to East Grinstead Queen Victoria Hospital for multiple surgeries. Having survived and become a Guinea Pig, he was authorised to return to operational flying once more. His luck finally ran out on 21 July 1944 when attacking Hamburg. Once again he was forced to parachute to safety but on this occasion he landed in water. He succumbed to drowning in the Elbe Estuary of the North Sea. His body was found washed ashore **6** weeks later by the crew of a German fishing boat. Despite Jack Calder appearing in the ranks of the wartime Guinea Pig Club committee and the indisputable evidence of having been a Guinea Pig, his name is absent from the Roll of Honour Board.

23,034

By July 1945, Leslie Irvin of the Irvin Airchute Company had enrolled this number of airmen into his Caterpillar Club. He had agreed to present a gold pin to every airman whose life was saved by one of his company's parachutes. In order to gain membership to his Caterpillar Club, prospective members were required to produce documentation of the incident to the parachute manufacturer. In many applications the parachutes were identified by serial numbers and types. Those details were frequently checked against the factory's production information as a form of integrity assurance. Letters to the parachute company were in some instances very detailed. The requirements for receiving a gold pin and club membership card were stringent. Each recipient of the Caterpillar Pin is living testimony to the lifesaving

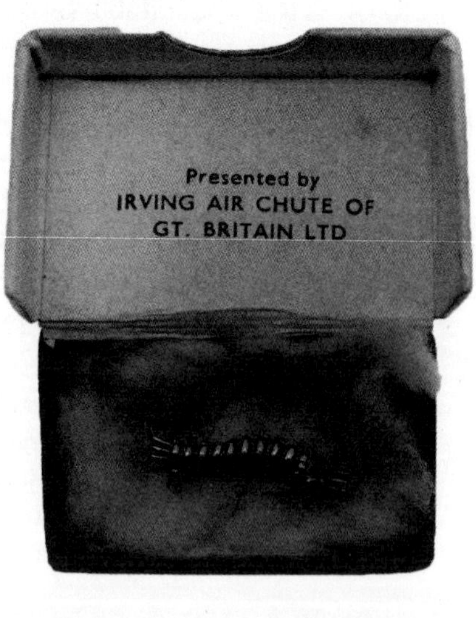

Irvin Parachute Caterpillar Club membership pin in the presentation box. Each small caterpillar pin was expertly hand engraved with the rank and name of the recipient. Many Guinea Pigs were entitled to apply for membership and receive a caterpillar pin following an emergency parachute escape.

ability of the Irvin Type Air Chute and a great many of Archibald McIndoe's patients owed their lives to the parachute before his medical expertise improved their lives. The statistics of Guinea Pigs who applied for and became members of Leslie Irvin's club is unknown.

500ft

The lowest height by which a Guinea Pig escaped flames by parachute belongs to the Canadian pilot Frank Hanton. On 17 July 1944, his Spitfire suffering from the loss of engine oil and coolant suddenly exploded in flames at around **500ft**. With his flying jacket alight and burning he escaped the cockpit but his parachute was only able to open at tree top height. Frank Hanton experienced an exceptionally hard impact hitting the ground. His facial burns had closed his eyes and he was unable to see. The Canadian pilot states that both Archibald McIndoe and Ross Tilley operated upon him, something which he was always indebted for throughout his remaining life.[110] Frank Hanton is amongst the few confirmed Guinea Pigs who successfully applied to join the Caterpillar Club .

58

Reginald Harrison arrived in England from Canada in July 1943. After his operational training he flew his first bombing operation on 15 March 1944. Returning home safely his Halifax bomber landed with a hung-up bomb which had not released properly over the target. The bomb dislodged as the heavy bomber touched the runway and it immediately exploded in the bomb bay. Harrison was blown out from the aircraft, receiving a flash burn to his left forearm as he was propelled by the blast. At the Queen Victoria Hospital, **58** pinch grafts were taken from his upper left leg and grafted to his arm. He recovered and returned to active operational flying. He experienced a further incident which enforced an emergency parachute escape over England on 9 August 1944.

1

Although few in numbers, a handful of Netherlanders who made their way to Britain after escaping the Nazis made a significant contribution flying with the Royal Air Force. Lieutenant Fritz Overeijnder is one identified Dutchman who operated within a Hudson aircraft which carried the Dutch nation's black-edged orange triangle insignia. On 8 March 1941, flying from Carew Cheriton in Pembrokeshire, his Lockheed Hudson aircraft T9356 named 'Brantas' crashed on the return flight. Fritz Overeijnder was seriously burnt and his aircraft was completely destroyed. Fritz holds the rare accolade of becoming the first of only **2** Dutch Guinea Pig Club members.

Fritz was permitted to resume flying with restricted duties within Transport Command.[111]

6 A broken or defective engine crank being used by Leading Aircraftsman Walter Cunningham at a South African flying school saw him fall into turning aircraft propellor blades on 15 April 1943. This was a most unfortunate accident, causing crippling injuries when both his hands were almost severed at the wrists, in addition to head injuries which in other circumstances would undoubtably have been fatal. His survival was remarkable and after a medical repatriation to England, Walter arrived at the Queen Victoria Hospital in May 1944. He received **6** surgical operations. Despite being inevitably absent at annual reunions, he was always most supportive to his fellow Guinea Pig Club members.[112]

2 On the morning of 16 August 1943, several Spitfire pilots intruded into occupied Europe actively seeking opportunistic targets. One Polish pilot, Sergeant Waclaw Korwel became engaged in an aerial dog fight of some ferocity with Luftwaffe fighters. The fuel tank of his Spitfire was hit and glass from the instruments in the cockpit shattered. He was also wounded in the left leg and had lost 2 entire fingers and a part of another finger. He managed to get his Spitfire back to the British shores where without landing gear he slewed into the ground near Brighton on the Sussex coast. At the Queen Victoria Hospital he underwent plastic surgery on his hands. Archibald McIndoe sought to restore as much mobility and dexterity as possible. Remarkably, Waclaw Korwel returned to combat flying and survived the war. This Polish Guinea Pig returned to his homeland where the subsequent Communist regime discriminated against him for his war service. On 24 March 1952, he was to lose his life to that persecution. The place of his burial still remains unknown. This brave Guinea Pig is recorded on the Roll of Honour as W. P. Korwell.

2 Nedim Erakdogam, and Karmel Intepe, Turkish Air Force officers, are the only known Turks to become Guinea Pigs. In 1940, the Turkish air brigades had the largest air force in the Balkans and the Middle East. The Turkish Armed Forces were prepared for war following the military alliance between neighbouring Bulgaria and the Axis Powers which was ratified in March 1941. The occupation of neighbouring Greece by those forces occurred in April 1941. Within a year, Turkey's borders were surrounded by German forces in the north-west and west, and Italian forces in the south-west. The

Turkish Air Force made daily reconnaissance flights over Bulgaria, Greece, the Greek Islands in the Aegean Sea, and the Dodecanese Islands which then belonged to Italy. During the war, Turkey sent pilots to the United Kingdom for training purposes. **14** pilots are known to have died, **1** of them shot down by a German intruder during a training flight in British air space. The rest died in numerous accidents. Turkey remained neutral until 23 February 1945, when they joined the Allies by themselves declaring war against Germany and Japan. Sixty-two days after that declaration, Nedim was flying as a passenger when a friendly fire incident took place which caused facial fractures and the loss of his right eye. This Turkish officer was transported to England and admitted to the care of Archibald McIndoe on 17 December 1945. Less is known of Karmel Intepe, as a Hurricane pilot he crashed into a tree sustaining facial injuries. He was treated at East Grinstead in 1945. In 1972, Intepe drove from Turkey to East Grinstead to attend the annual reunion. He did so because he held the desire to offer his gratitude to those who had cared for him.

140

Australian fighter pilot Ronald Adcock flew several operations attacking the V1 Flying Bombs in 1944. An Australian news release announced he had been successful in shooting down three and had attained **140** operational sorties against many targets. These included **33** locomotives, **25** river barges and **30** train carriages. He flew Typhoons and later converted to fly the Tempest fighter in 1945. He may well be the only Guinea Pig to have joined the club flying that exceptional aircraft which was capable of flying at over **400** miles an hour. Flying over Germany at Hildeshiem on 13 February 1945, he was shot down and received burns to his hands and face and a damaged shoulder before escaping by parachute. He became a prisoner of war. When released, he was admitted to the care of Archibald McIndoe on 30 April 1945.[113]

4

Robert Nixon Dalkin enlisted in the Royal Australian Air Force on 8 January 1940, and was commissioned shortly thereafter. He initially flew the Lockheed Hudson light bombers on reconnaissance duties protecting the Australian coastline. In January 1942, Dalkin became a flight commander at Darwin where he flew numerous strikes against Japanese targets. On 30 June 1942, he led **4** aircraft on a night attack upon Timor in which **8** enemy aircraft were probably destroyed. Dalkin was awarded the Distinguished Flying Cross.[114] The citation commended his leadership and courage in the face of heavy anti-aircraft fire against Japanese targets. In 1944, he was attached to the Royal Air Force Bomber Command in Britain to develop techniques that could possibly be adopted in the Pacific war against the Japanese. He flew operations over occupied Europe as an Australian Wing Commander and survived unscathed. On 9 May 1944, he was walking in the blackout when he fell into an uncovered hole sustaining lacerations to his leg. No further details are known apart from his admittance to a station sick quarter and his subsequent transfer to the Queen Victoria Hospital on 29 May 1944. Undoubtedly, Robert Dalkin became the club's highest ranking Australian, but in most unusual circumstances.

6

The Fleet Air Arm's second Guinea Pig was Navy pilot Eric Pearce. He was serving in an air-sea rescue squadron in 1945. On 1 May at Lee-on-Solent, he took a Sea Otter seaplane into the air for a test flight and a connecting rod in the engine broke on take-off. This induced a headlong crash into the shingle bank. The engine came loose in the accident and it fell onto the pilots' cabin where Pearce was sitting. He was pulled from the wreckage by a Naval Surgeon and taken to the Royal Hospital Haslar where he remained unconscious for **6** weeks. The date of his admission into Archibald McIndoe's care is unknown as are the operations undertaken. The engine had crushed his face and led to the loss of one eye.[115]

1

On 15 April 1945, Canadian Guinea Pig Norman McHolm was taken on a flight to view the ruins of central Germany. Norman had previously received surgery at East Grinstead to his nose and herniated back discs after a flying accident on 8 November 1944. He had experienced a dramatic accident with a failed take off in a Halifax heavy bomber ending up with insufficient runway. His aircraft slewed across countryside and ended up in a drainage ditch. His nose was almost torn away and he sustained several significant crush injuries. His initial hospital had been the Royal Navy Hospital at Kingseat, Aberdeen before being transported to the Queen Victoria Hospital on 20 December 1944.[116]

2

The Canadian pilot John Hughes whose wife designed the Guinea Pig Club badge, sought the assistance of surgery to both of his ears in January 1945. It is unclear if the disproportionate protruding of ear tissue caused difficulties for flying safety or otherwise. Regardless of those unknown circumstance, both ears were adjusted by surgery and John was welcomed into the Guinea Pig Club. This may well be one of the most unusual circumstances of membership but being allowed to wear the Guinea Pig Club badge designed by his wife no doubt made for a distinctly proud pair of individuals who appear to have supported the club at any opportunity.

128 The Canadian navigator Hans Raymond Anderson with his British pilot Gordon Ayton took off for an Atlantic transit ferry flight in a Mosquito aircraft in June 1945. The end of the war had resulted in a surplus of new military aircraft, and their Mosquito had been built by De Havilland at Downsview, Ontario. It was on the first stage of an onwards delivery flight from Canada to the United Kingdom. Following the first transit, the aircraft had taken off on 28 June from Greenland, to fly to Prestwick Airport, Scotland. It was over Ireland, probably diverted by weather conditions, in failing light when the Mosquito was required to force land in a field as fuel was diminishing. The aircraft careered across open land in Galway Ireland into a stone wall where it burst into flames. Anderson was rescued but the pilot was killed. Hans Anderson was given treatment at St Endas Military Hospital. He had sustained injuries to both arms and burns to his buttocks.[117] He arrived at the Queen Victoria Hospital on 2 September 1945. **3** surgeries took place. The *Belfast Telegraph* carried the following story on 30 June 1945: 'EIRE PLANE CRASH. A Mosquito aeroplane of the Royal Canadian Air Force crashed in Co. Galway shortly after midnight (British time) on Thursday, and Pilot Officer Gordon Ayton was burned to death and Flight Lieut. H. W. Anderson severely burned. They were the only occupants of the aeroplane. The aeroplane developed engine trouble over Galway Bay, but managed to fly over Galway city before it fell on low-lying land. Firemen and members of the L.D.F. extricated Anderson from the burning aeroplane but were unable to reach Ayton whose body was recovered later. The aeroplane was flying from Greenland to Scotland.' The deceased pilot Gordon Ayton had completed **128** operational sorties over **3** tours of duty and was the holder of the Distinguished Flying Cross.

1945 The Guinea Pig Club became an officially registered charity in July 1945.

Chapter 4

A Legacy – The Guinea Pig Club and its Members after the War

1 Geoffrey Page's book *Tale of a Guinea Pig* was dedicated by him to McIndoe with the words. 'To Archie McIndoe whose surgeon's fingers gave me back my pilot's hands'.[1]

298 On 11 August 1945, the *Horsham Times Sussex and Surrey Courier* published that the Guinea Pig Club had this number of members.

1945 Victory in the European war celebrations was welcomed within the hospital. The Guinea Pig club remained deeply embedded in the system of care to those who continued to occupy the operating theatres and wards. A legacy had already been built, and it continued to deliver for over **60** years. The immediate post-war period saw the hospital accept patients who by various privations had been prevented from specialist medical treatment. The previously

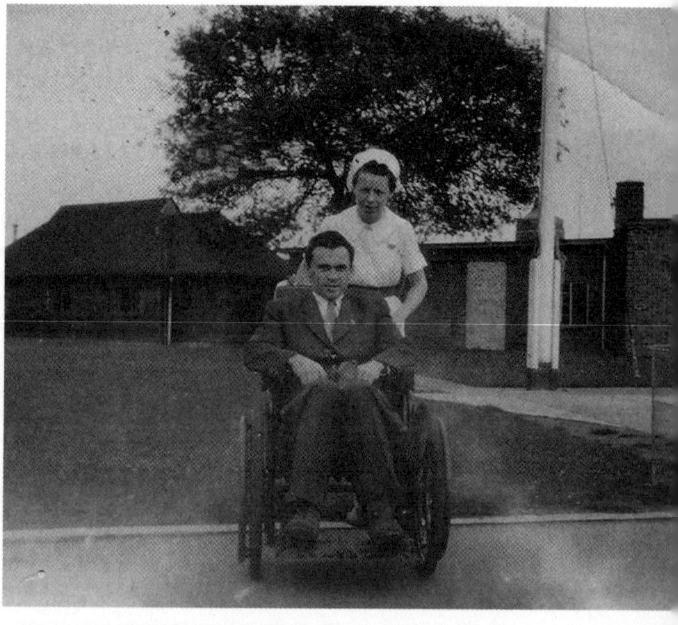

Alois Siska in his wheelchair wearing civilian clothing with his nurse. Seen in the hospital grounds providing a view of the buildings and the hospital flagpole. (*Free Czechoslovak Air Force Associates Ltd. Dagmar Siskova-Johnson collection*)

mentioned Czechoslovakian, Alois Siska, is an example of an airman who had experienced imprisonment in Colditz Castle. He arrived at East Grinstead in June **1945**. The war in the Far East continued with great ferocity whilst the destruction across Europe was contemplated and assessed.

1 The Royal Canadian Air Force flag was lowered from the Queen Victoria Hospital flag pole on Wednesday 5 September 1945. The Canadian Wing Hospital facility was officially handed over to the Chairman of the Hospital, Edward Blount OBE. The Canadian Hospital Detachment of staff held a farewell dinner and dance which took place at the Rainbow Ballroom at the Whitehall in the evening.

6 The number of operations at the Queen Victoria Hospital that awaited Aircraftsman Anthony Allard who was injured in a crash at Hullavington in Wiltshire on 7 September 1945. Allard had graduated as an apprentice from Halton. He was amongst four ex-apprentices who had been rewarded with an air experience flight in an Avro Lancaster. The aircraft crashed with Tony Allard being thrown clear. He went back into the burning wreckage to try to save his colleagues but was unable to do so. He was the only survivor but

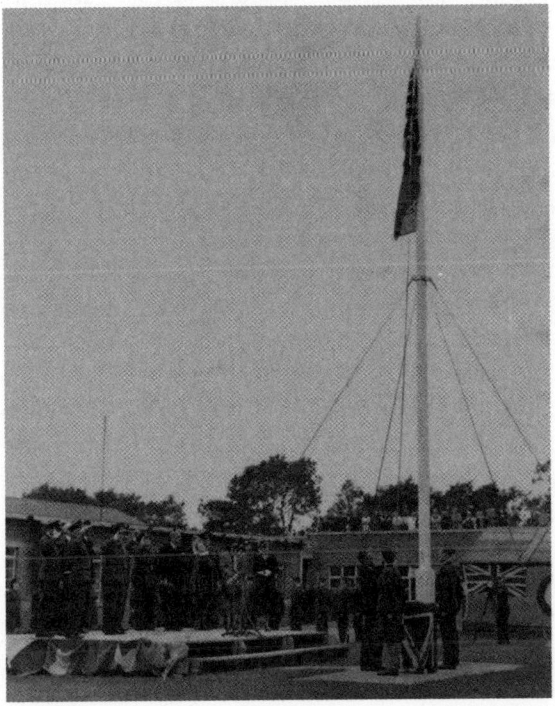

The lowering of the Canadian flag initiating the official handing over of the Canadian Wing building. The building was given over fully to Queen Victoria Hospital in the flag-lowering ceremony in September 1945. (*Canadian Weekly* 14.9.45.)

badly burned and spent a long time in the burns unit at Cosford. He was later admitted at East Grinstead on 4 February 1946. A romance took place with nurse Sylvia Syvret whom he later married on 25 June 1949.

1 The Canadian war artist Charles Goldhamer painted many watercolours and drew images of patients and scenes within the Canadian Wing on and around 18 September 1945.

1 Group Captain Ross Tilley departed the hospital on 23 September 1945, embarking for Canada on the SS *New Amsterdam* at Southampton Docks.

£7 The Forest Row Victory Celebration Committee donated this sum to the Guinea Pig Club on 29 September 1945.

110,600 The number of pilots trained on behalf of the Royal Air Force within **9** different countries during the Second World War.[2] The Guinea Pig Club records establish that just **193** pilots from that total became Guinea Pigs.[3]

1 The King's first post-war Christmas message to the nation in December 1945 was immediately followed by a live broadcast direct from the Ward Three Christmas party at East Grinstead Hospital. The BBC announcer reported, 'Of all the hospitals in this country, the Queen Victoria is world famed and airmen of all nations have found rest, peace and healing there'. Archibald McIndoe spoke and ended with the plea that the public should not forget these boys who come to us here at East Grinstead from all over the world.[4]

1 Tom Gleave served as the clubs' **1st** and only honorary Chief Guinea Pig until his death in 1993.

1 One Guinea Pig attended the Nuremburg War Trials held in Germany between 20 November 1945 to 1 October 1946. Robert Wright had commenced his war as Aide-de-Camp to Air Marshal Sir Hugh Dowding, Commander-in-Chief of Fighter Command between July and October 1940. Wright continued in that duty under Sholto Douglas, Dowding's successor. It was in November 1944, whilst serving as a radar operator in a Mosquito that Robert joined the Guinea Pig Club. During a landing approach with a faulty engine, the second engine stalled and the aircraft crashed and burst into flames.

Robert Wright was pulled from the flames by Corporal Thomas Charles Woodhead who was awarded the British Empire Medal for his bravery. The recommendation for that award explains further: 'One afternoon in November, 1944, an aircraft, whilst attempting to make a forced landing on an airfield, crashed and burst into flames. Corporal Woodhead who was working in the vicinity ran to the scene of the accident in company with other airmen. By the time they arrived one wing was burning fiercely and the fire was spreading to the cockpit and fuselage. Disregarding the flames and the ammunition which had started to explode, Corporal Woodhead and his helpers jumped on to the port wing and the cockpit Perspex canopy and tried to break into the cockpit but they were unable to release the emergency roof exit or to get at the crew. They could see that the pilot was bent over the control column and that the

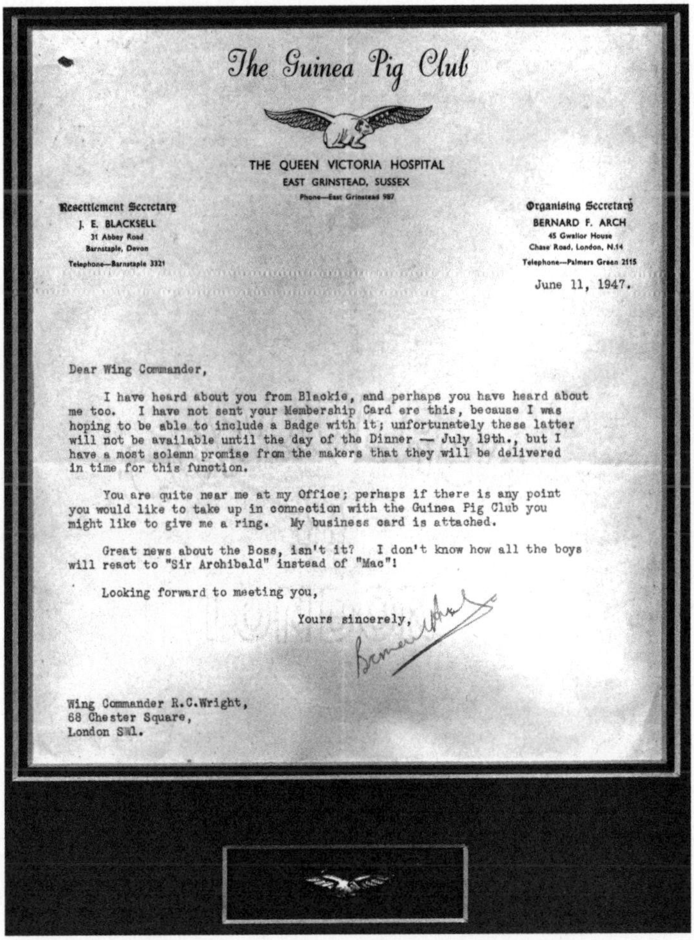

The Guinea Pig Club

THE QUEEN VICTORIA HOSPITAL
EAST GRINSTEAD, SUSSEX
Phone—East Grinstead 987

Resettlement Secretary
J. E. BLACKSELL
31 Abbey Road
Barnstaple, Devon
Telephone—Barnstaple 3321

Organising Secretary
BERNARD F. ARCH
45 Gwalior House
Chase Road, London, N.14
Telephone—Palmers Green 2115

June 11, 1947.

Dear Wing Commander,

I have heard about you from Blackie, and perhaps you have heard about me too. I have not sent your Membership Card ere this, because I was hoping to be able to include a Badge with it; unfortunately these latter will not be available until the day of the Dinner — July 19th., but I have a most solemn promise from the makers that they will be delivered in time for this function.

You are quite near me at my Office; perhaps if there is any point you would like to take up in connection with the Guinea Pig Club you might like to give me a ring. My business card is attached.

Great news about the Boss, isn't it? I don't know how all the boys will react to "Sir Archibald" instead of "Mac"!

Looking forward to meeting you,

Yours sincerely,

Bernard Arch

Wing Commander R.C.Wright,
68 Chester Square,
London S.W.1.

Guinea Pig Club letter sent from the club secretary in 1947 to Wing Commander Robert Wright concerning his badge and membership.

navigator was on the floor. By this time a fire engine had arrived and commenced to play foam jets onto the cockpit, but the heat had become so intense that all were forced to retire. A few moments later the navigator's head and shoulders appeared through a hole which had been made in the side of the fuselage [Robert Wright]. Despite the intense heat and danger from exploding tanks, Corporal Woodhead immediately dashed into the flames and dragged the injured man to safety. Corporal Woodhead then attempted to return and search for the pilot but was driven back by the heat which was by then too great to allow of any further rescue attempt to be made. Corporal Woodhead had shown complete disregard of his personal safety and his action in finally rescuing the navigator from the blazing wreckage was one requiring great courage.' Wright was treated at Ely Hospital before being transferred to the care of Archibald McIndoe. After his recovery and during his convalescence Wright was readmitted at East Grinstead a second time when a V2 rocket exploded close to his house.[5] Following his attendance at the Nuremburg War Trials, Wright subsequently worked as an advisor on the Battle of Britain movie and wrote several books.

2 Guinea Pig Robert Wright became the official biographer of two senior RAF commanders of the Second World War, Hugh Dowding and Sholto Douglas after the war.[6]

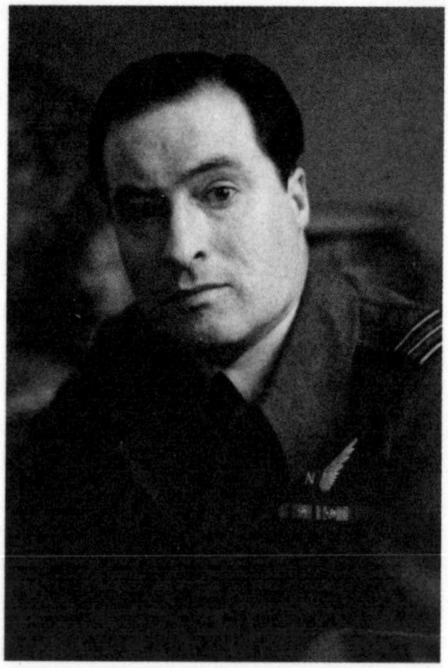

Wing Commander Bob Wright wearing his battledress flying tunic supporting his navigator wing and medal ribbons. Wright resigned his commission in the RAF in late 1947, becoming a successful writer and historian.

2 Surgeons Sir Archibald McIndoe and Jerry Moore from the Queen Victoria Hospital were invited to the French Embassy in London in May 1950. The French Ambassador presented the French decoration of Commander of the Legion of Honour to McIndoe. The citation for the Commander of the Legion of Honour read: 'During the war of 1939-45, he founded and organised to the profit of the Allied Forces, the East Grinstead Plastic Surgery Centre, and has thus enabled many disfigured French servicemen to return to their normal lives after long and difficult treatments which demanded the greatest care in every detail and which brought into play the highest qualities required of a surgeon. He displayed true genius in his operations and has obtained the most prodigious results. Since the founding of the plastic surgery centre, he has shown an untiring devotion and boundless energy. By making possible for many French servicemen a life which otherwise would have been indeed difficult, Sir Archibald McIndoe deserves the recognition of the French Army.'

Moore received the Officer of the Legion. The citation for the Officer of the Legion for Jerry Moore reads: '... He attended many French servicemen who were wounded in the face and limbs and thanks to the high standard of his efficiency, his devotion and unceasing efforts, he has achieved results which are quite remarkable. By thus giving back a desire for life to the French wounded and totally disfigured, he has merited the recognition of the French Air Force.'

11 The number of titles held by Archibald McIndoe, including medical qualifications and military recognition from grateful allies who acknowledged the saving of many lives. In descending order of attainment, they were:

Honours – Fellow of the Royal College of Surgeons 1948.

Knighthood 1947 – Knight Commander of the Most Excellent Order of the British Empire.

CBE 1944 – Commander of the Most Excellent Order of the British Empire.

Commander Legion of Honour – The highest French order of merit, both military and civil.

Commander Order of the White Lion – (Czechoslovakia). The Order of the White Lion became an award to those who had helped liberate Czechoslovakia from occupation by Nazi Germany. Following the surrender of Germany in May 1945, a large number of foreign bestowals were made by presenting the Order of the White Lion to senior officers of the Allied militaries.

Officer Order of Polonia Restituta 1945 – The Polish state order was conferred on both military and civilians as well as on foreigners for outstanding achievements. It is Poland's second-highest civilian state award.

Commander Order of Orange Nassau – The Dutch order of chivalry for recipients who have distinguished themselves by outstanding or extremely important work or have rendered service of international or even global importance.

Fellow – American College of Surgeons 1934.

Postgraduate diploma and Fellow – The Royal College of Surgeons 1932.

Bachelor of Medicine – Bachelor of Surgery degree (New Zealand) 1923.

1946

The Guinea Pig Club accepted into its membership the Fleet Air Arm pilot John Pelly on 25 April 1946. A rare Royal Navy Guinea Pig, Pelly had crashed on the aircraft carrier HMS *Theseus* and suffered burns to his back, legs and hands. Pelly had been given the instruction to cut his engine by the landing controller on the aircraft carrier. He was not happy with his position and thrust the throttle of his 816 Squadron Firefly aircraft fully open. The result saw him crashing in the bridge structure of the ship. The aircraft broke its back in the observer's cockpit and had an observer been flying with him, he would have been killed. Miraculously, John was thrown out of the aircraft and recovered from the sea badly injured.[7]

1

After the war, Archibald McIndoe invited fellow surgeon Fenton Braithwaite working at Rauceby Hospital to join the East Grinstead medical team. It is assumed that he resigned his commission in the Royal Air Force to do so. His previous experience at Rauceby and then at East Grinstead enabled him to publish a paper demonstrating the importance of blood transfusion in the management of severely burned patients and thereafter on the anatomical changes in the blood supply of the skin in tube pedicles.

£87,000

On 25 July 1946, the American Wing Surgical Centre was officially opened at the Queen Victoria Hospital by the hospital's patron, Queen Elizabeth. The American Wing contained five operating theatres and a library amongst other facilities. It was built largely from the generosity of the British War Relief Society of America, under its president, Mr Clark Minor. Additionally, a gift of **£87,000** had been made, thanks to the influence of Mr Kelsey Fry and Mr Le Crohn of the London Dental Society. Further money from the war organisations of the British Red Cross Society and the Order of

St John of Jerusalem was contributed for the actual building and provision of an X ray unit.

16 The number of nationalities stated extant in the Queen Victoria Hospital's Guinea Pig Club. This figure was quoted by Archibald McIndoe and Mr Blacksell reporting to the Royal Air Force Benevolent Fund in 1956.[8]

360 Cuthbert was a retired Bomber Command carrier pigeon who, having been slightly injured over Duisburg in 1943, came under the care of the Guinea Pig family. His presence was notified to the wider Guinea Pig audience in the club's newsletter of 1949. It is unclear exactly who cared for Cuthbert. Every Bomber Station had a 'pigeon keeper' who came under the command of the Station Signals Officer.[9] Each bird was registered and by example, pigeon NU.42E8554 was released by the crew of Lancaster ED717 who ditched on 14 April 1943. The crew were at a position of some **360** miles from their station. The pigeon flew for **8** hours and **30** minutes carrying the message of distress which was successfully received. The crew were rescued.

10 Ray Leupp was an American volunteer who flew Hurricane fighters for the Royal Canadian Air Force. Ray had become a Guinea Pig following his treatment for his smashed face in an accident in July 1943. Hitting the instrument panel also caused the loss of an eye. He was admitted to the Queen Victoria Hospital within **10** days of the crash. He rehabilitated at Marchwood Park between his operations. Ray Leupp spent his time studying for veterinary qualifications. Overcoming the loss of his eye, he qualified as a vet and practised in Ohio. This American Guinea Pig was a consistent communicator and contributor to the Guinea Pig Club newsletters throughout his life. The naming of his practice, the Marchwood Animal Hospital was clearly influenced by his memories of his rehabilitation.[10]

28 The first **28** issues of the Guinea Pig Club newsletter were printed with a coloured ink front cover page with the illustrative 'Two Types' bandaged Guinea Pig artwork created by Henry Standen.

1946 The Guinea Pig Club badge described in the newsletters as 'Pig Couchant' describes the guinea pig as standing on all fours between a pair of wings. It was a pressed metal badge fitted with a pin fastener. This design became the recognised Guinea Pig Club official membership lapel badge and appeared on letter headings. The

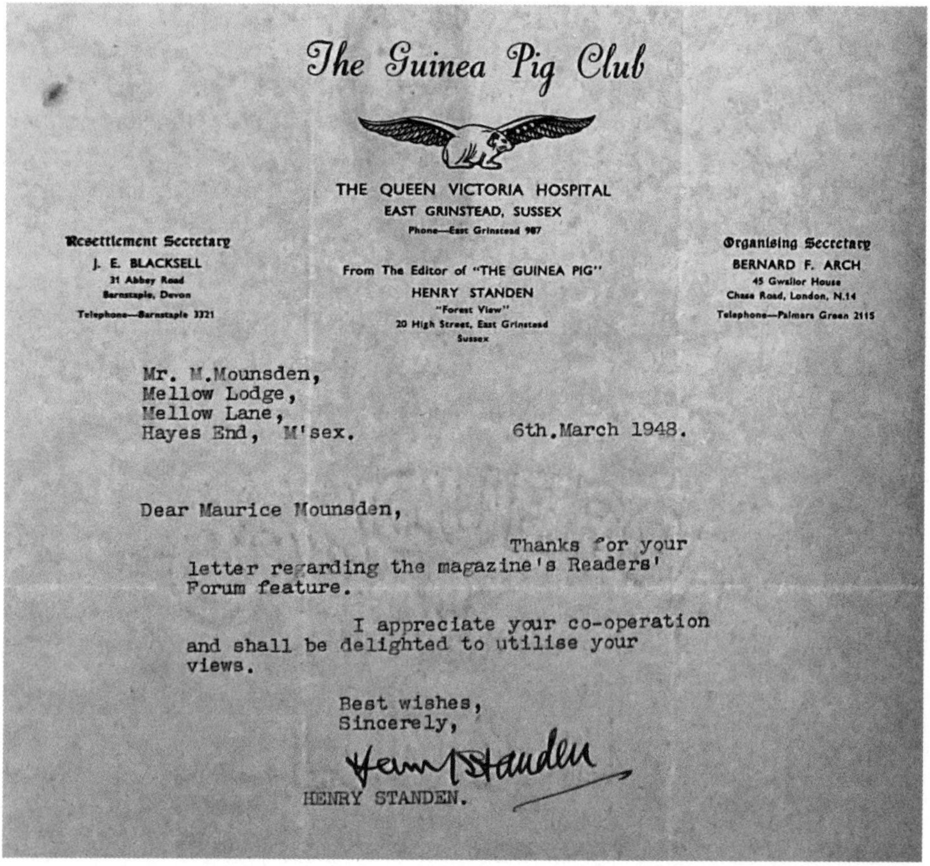

The Guinea Pig Club

THE QUEEN VICTORIA HOSPITAL
EAST GRINSTEAD, SUSSEX
Phone—East Grinstead 987

Resettlement Secretary
J. E. BLACKSELL
31 Abbey Road
Barnstaple, Devon
Telephone—Barnstaple 3321

From The Editor of "THE GUINEA PIG"
HENRY STANDEN
"Forest View"
20 High Street, East Grinstead
Sussex

Organising Secretary
BERNARD F. ARCH
45 Gwalior House
Chase Road, London, N.14
Telephone—Palmers Green 2115

Mr. M.Mounsden,
Mellow Lodge,
Mellow Lane,
Hayes End, M'sex.

6th.March 1948.

Dear Maurice Mounsden,

Thanks for your letter regarding the magazine's Readers' Forum feature.

I appreciate your co-operation and shall be delighted to utilise your views.

Best wishes,
Sincerely,

Henry Standen

HENRY STANDEN.

Guinea Pig Club letter sent to Maurice Mounsden by Henry Standen in 1948. The magazine editor and cartoonist thanking Maurice for a suggestion over matters relating to what had been a proposal for a readers' forum in the Guinea Pig magazine.

design of the new badge was credited to Mrs John Hughes, wife of Canadian Guinea Pig Flying Officer Hughes. It was fully adopted from **1946** onwards. In **1949**, a less ostentatiously sized badge, replicating the same design with pin fitting was commissioned to be worn as a tie-pin or lapel emblem. This badge was no more than a third the size of the original.

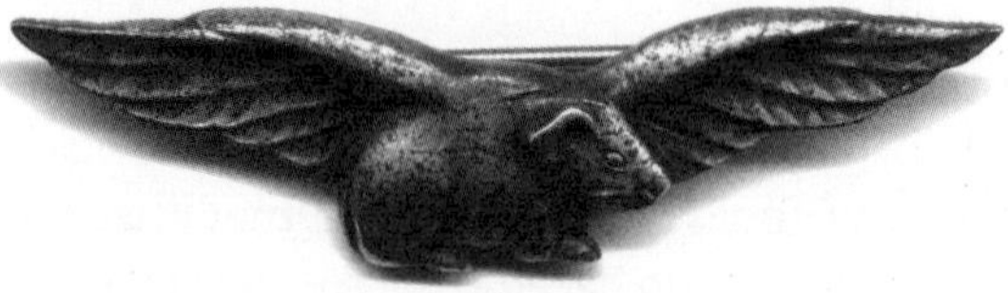

Guinea Pig Club metal membership badge.

2 Not all Guinea Pig records exist, for example there are cases where patients are unable to be properly identified. The names A. Stansburg and M. Szafranski are **2** recognised Guinea Pigs on the Roll of Honour where no identities can be attributed. Likewise, **5** men, B. Owen-Smith, F. H. Mahn, J. P. Calder, G. Shaughnessy and H. Avery are missing names upon the Roll of Honour board but regarded as Guinea Pigs.

3 Three Guinea Pigs, Jack Alloway, Bill Foxley and Frederick Rix, took advantage of the opportunity of a sponsored recuperation trip to Switzerland in 1946. They were accompanied by Claude Allen. The group were invited to meet Winston Churchill whilst he holidayed nearby at Villa Choisi, a property now regarded as being of national significance to Switzerland. Several of Winston's landscape paintings were composed from that particular location which Churchill very much favoured.

1 Henry Standen, distributed *The Guinea Pig* magazine worldwide. It appears Winston Churchill was also a recipient and in appreciation, Churchill sent Henry an autographed copy of one of his own books..[11]

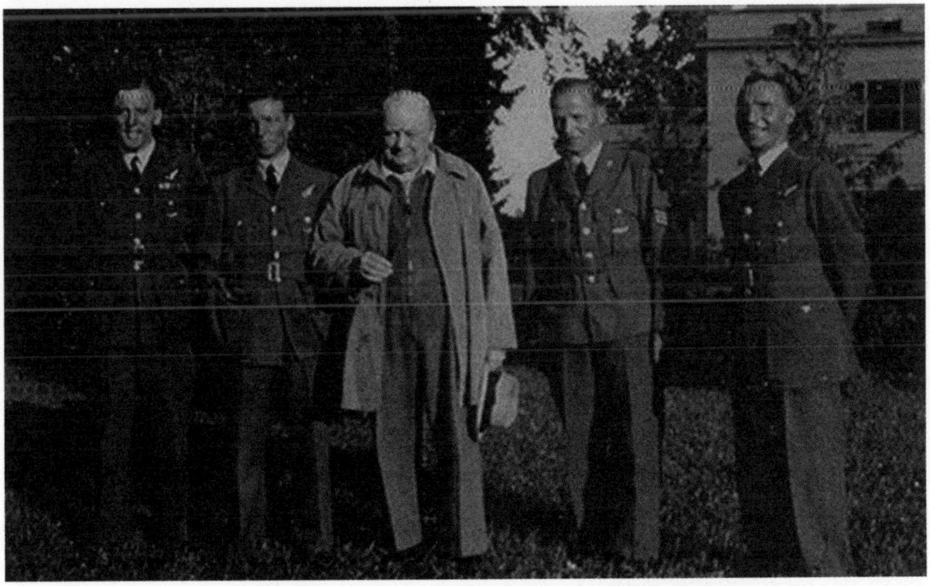

The Guinea Pigs with Winson Churchill in Switzerland, an image often wrongly attributed to have been photographed at the hospital in East Grinstead. Jack Alloway first left, Bill Foxley second left, Fred Rix far right. Claud Allen is wearing a Sergeant's tunic without a wing brevet suggesting he may well have been a medical orderly. Three group were invited to meet Winston Churchill whilst he holidayed and painted at Villa Choisi.

11

South African Bernard Levin was transferred to the care of Archibald McIndoe in April 1946. His injuries must have been severe as the records indicate **11** operations were undertaken at the Queen Victoria Hospital. He had been flying on 6 June 1944 at Bulawayo in Southern Rhodesia when an accident took place, and an ensuing fire caused facial and hand injuries which were treated in his home country. Circumstances thereafter unusually saw the South African transported to England and **2** years after his accident, he became a Guinea Pig.

7

The number of operations undertaken by Sir Archibald McIndoe upon George Reynolds. George had served as a pilot in Bomber Command but natural causes induced the need of surgery to a neoplasm tumour of his jaw. Operated upon in June 1946, McIndoe's surgery was most effective and it provided **7** years of good health. In 1953, he was readmitted at East Grinstead as the tumour had returned aggressively. George subsequently died whilst in the care of McIndoe. The impression he had cast upon Archibald McIndoe was such that he penned an appreciation to his life in the April 1954 Guinea Pig newsletter.

1947

On 10 May that year, Winston Churchill was presented with the French military honour the Medaille Militaire at the Cour des Invalides in Paris. Just days before this event, Churchill had entertained several Guinea Pig Club members at his home Chartwell in Mapleton Road, Westerham, Kent.

50

It was reported that in June 1947 there were **50** Guinea Pigs under treatment at the Queen Victoria Hospital.[12]

1947

In December that year notices appeared in the press informing former Servicemen how to claim their medals. The Government required war veterans to apply for the medals using a postcard available at any Post Office from Monday, 31 May 1948. The forms were colour coded. The army forms were printed with black ink, Royal Air Force with light blue ink and the Navy used green ink. There appear to be no comments published in the Guinea Pig magazine upon this subject.

1948

The second contingent of Guinea Pig Club members departed for a Swiss recuperation holiday on 11 May that year. Amongst them was Raymond Henry Brooke, who had endured **35** operations being

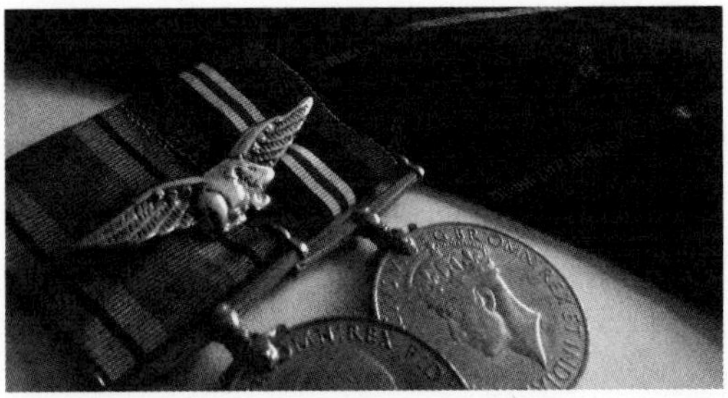

The medal group of Flight Mechanic John Hill. On 25 March 1945, Warrant Officer Thompson was flying a Typhoon which crashed into the crew room of a dispersal hut on the airfield at Aston Down. The aircraft crashed and exploded in flames. Five ground crew were killed, Flight Mechanic John Hill was amongst the **18** people admitted to hospital with terrible burn injuries. He was immediately transferred to Cosford Hospital for specialist treatment which progressed with admittance into the Queen Victoria Hospital where he became a Guinea Pig. John Hill and his twin sister eventually emigrated to Australia but remained in contact throughout his life communicating by letter to the Guinea Pig magazine.

rebuilt after suffering deep penetrating burns. Brooke had been off duty in the local cafe at Freckleton, Lancashire. A Liberator was on a test flight and got caught in storm clouds; the pilot lost control, crashing in the centre of Freckleton, demolishing three houses and the cafe. The area was strewn in aviation fuel which ignited. The crash also took out the infant wing of Freckleton Holy Trinity School, where a class was in session, killing **38** of the **41** students aged between four to six, and a number of adults. Raymond Brooke received burns to his face, hands, and right leg and received treatment at East Grinstead hospital for the next **5** years.[13]

1

A civilian became a rare Guinea Pig Club member by appointment as an 'Honorary Member' in the immediate post-war period. Clifford Stone had been a civilian, interned by the Japanese military forces. He had suffered injuries which are not readily identified. However, after victory was achieved against the Japanese, persons unknown saw the condition of Clifford and his injuries and arrangements were put in place for his transfer to the Queen Victoria Hospital for reconstructive surgery. Whilst in Sussex, he involved himself in Guinea Pig Club activities. He was the only Chinese member to become an honorary member. Clifford returned to China. He certainly survived adversity on more than one occasion in his lifetime.[14]

4

The number of years that passed between an accident and eventual surgery at the Queen Victoria Hospital for South African student pilot, John Nivison. He was flying a Tiger Moth on 21 December 1943 when he crashed. The ensuing fire caused burns to his shoulders, arms and hands. Medical treatment in South Africa was provided. **4** years after the accident the South African was admitted to the care of Archibald McIndoe on 23 January 1948. He underwent **4** operations and became a Guinea Pig.

1 A Czechoslovakian Guinea Pig Club member, Karel Snadjr became employed as a stone carver for the Imperial War Graves Commission. Clearly his injuries did not prevent him delivering the skill required to set the names of those who had given their lives to attain victory in both World Wars. Headstones are inscribed with the details of the individual, including name, rank, awards, service number, religious emblem and often at the base a personal inscription provided by the family.

2 In October 1946, Jill Mullins and Archibald McIndoe toured medical hospitals in America. The prestige of the work carried out at the Queen Victoria Hospital had preceded them. Film stars and celebrities greeted them, including Ava Gardner who was to become one of McIndoe's private patients. Their meeting created a trusting partnership. 'The Ava Gardner Trust' was a legacy of generosity and

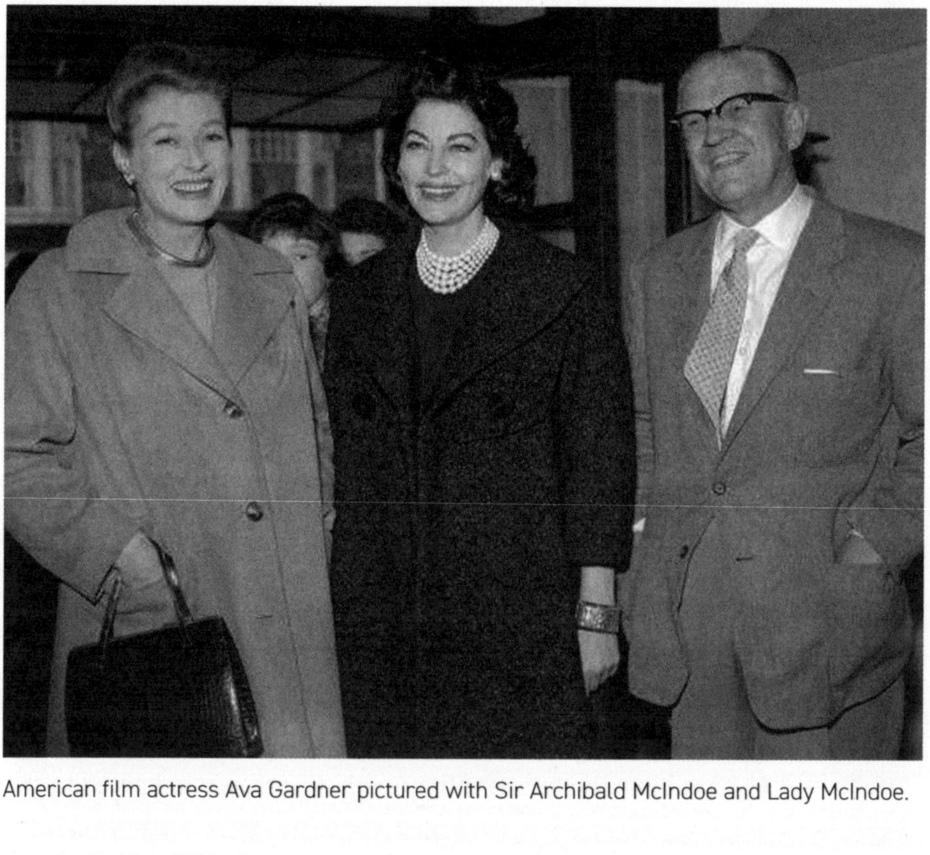

American film actress Ava Gardner pictured with Sir Archibald McIndoe and Lady McIndoe.

compassion instigated by Ava, it later became her living trust in which The Queen Victoria Hospital Foundation Trust was identified in legal terms as a beneficiary. Ava selected the Queen Victoria Hospital Foundation Trust because Archibald McIndoe had treated her after a fall from a horse at the Peralta ranch in Spain in October of 1957. In recovering from the fall, Ava became more and more involved with The Guinea Pig Club. In her autobiography, *Ava My Story*, she said: 'I met a lot of them and we danced and laughed together. They were so brave I could have wept. Archie told me my visits did them a lot of good, but I'm sure they helped me more than I ever helped them.'[15]

1947 The 'Friends of the Guinea Pig Club' badge was an elaborate design incorporating a light blue enamel filling upon the metal backed badge. The gilt flying Guinea Pig symbol was present with the letters F.G.P.C. underneath. The small golden guinea pig was half-surrounded with laurel leaves. This badge was sparingly awarded. The 1980s saw another 'Friends' badge designed and produced by Pilgrim Trophies which symbolically referenced a traditional Guinea Pig mammal, far removed from the elegant original badge.

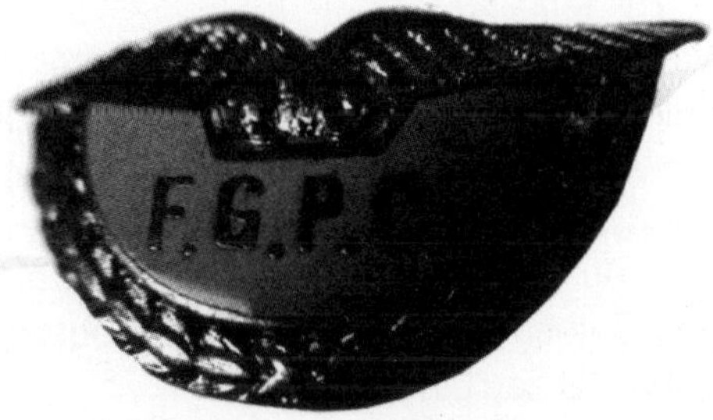

Friends of the Guinea Pig Club badge.

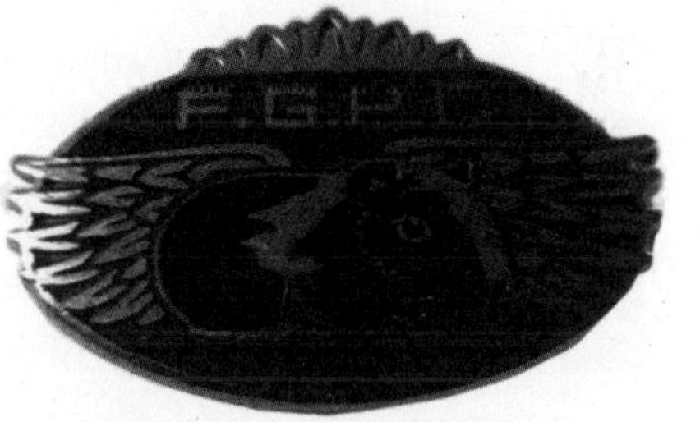

The later Friends of the Guinea Pig Club badge.

40 On 20 November 1946, **40** surgeons including McIndoe agreed to form the British Association of Plastic Surgeons.

1947 The post-war restriction on paper supplies eased in that year and it was proposed that the Guinea Pig Club newsletter could now be printed and distributed three times per annum. This was never achieved.

6 The **6th** annual dinner at East Grinstead took place on 19 July 1947. The prior annual general meeting held in the hospital's American

Wing lecture room was filmed by Pathe News as the Guinea Pigs congregated outside the main building. Cinemagoers across Britain saw the footage on their screens in the following weeks.

1

One official Guinea Pig Club membership badge was by request, provided to the curator of the Imperial War Museum in London in 1947.

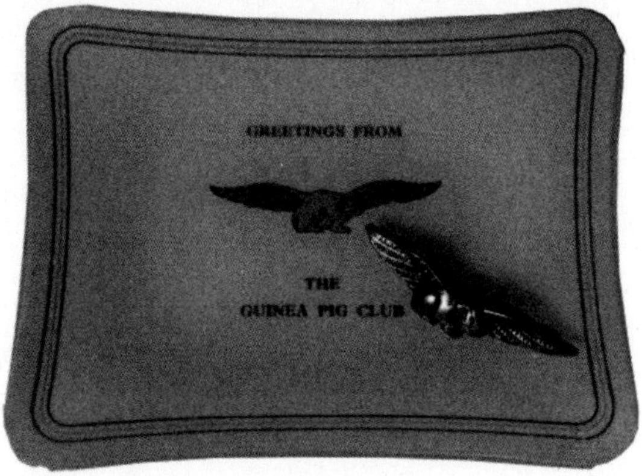

Guinea Pig Club badge and glass pin tray.

230

The number of Guinea Pigs who attended the official annual dinner at the Whitehall in East Grinstead on their 6th anniversary dinner. The guest of honour at that event was Marshal of the RAF Lord Portal.

20th

Sir Archibald McIndoe flew to Africa on 20 July 1947. During his visit he met amongst others, Guinea Pig club members Godfrey Edmonds, Graham Lawson and Barney Levin.

0

Zero – The proud statistic of Sister Meally of Ward Three at East Grinstead who unashamedly recorded that no patients lost their life in her care.

2

The number of camels owned by Flight Lieutenant Mohammed El Demerdash of the Egyptian Air Force who in February 1947, added to the various nationalities who had been admitted to the Queen Victoria Hospital. Insufficient records exist to establish his actual injuries or the medical expertise provided to him.

1

Keith Base is the only Guinea Pig who can claim to become a member after firing rockets from a Spitfire. On 2 May 1947, he was

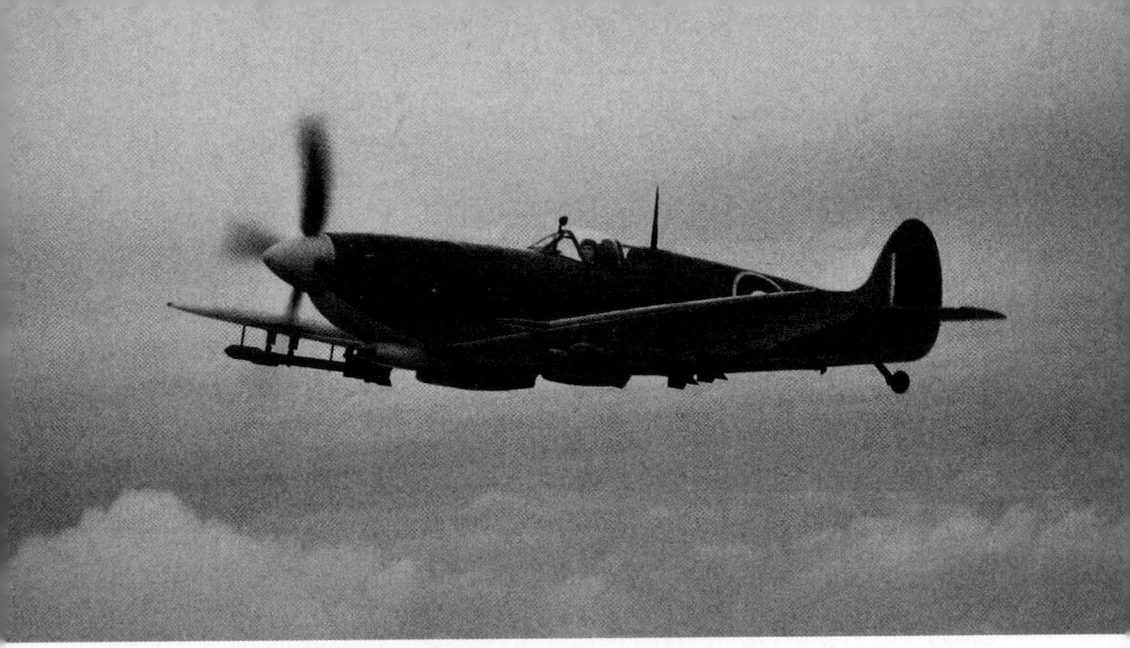

Spitfire flown by Guinea Pig Keith Base.

test-firing rockets at Little Rissington in Gloucestershire. The firing had no effect upon his Spitfire but when his engine malfunctioned, it enforced an emergency wheel-up landing. Keith smashed his face onto the gyroscope gunsight, becoming somewhat disfigured with lacerations. After treatment at the Rauceby hospital, he was moved to the care of Archibald McIndoe at East Grinstead. His injuries led to him being invalided out of the RAF in 1950.[16]

12 The Royal Air Force Benevolent Fund donated £4,000 to the Guinea Pig Club in 1948. This was distributed between 12 recipients after assessing each as in need of financial assistance..[17]

4 Morris Motors Limited allocated one 8-horsepower car per quarter to the Guinea Pig Club during 1948. It appears no records exist as to who the **4** recipients of this generous gift were.

325 The number of Guinea Pigs invited to attend the **7th** annual dinner on 4 September 1948 at the Whitehall. The Belgium Grape export company presented each table of attendees with a bunch of grapes with a message. 'In Remembrance of the Liberation of the Nursery district – 4 September 1948'.

15 Sir Archibald McIndoe announced in September 1948 that there were this number of Guinea Pigs still receiving treatment and care in the Queen Victoria hospital. The operating schedule anticipated that those patients would hopefully complete their medical care within **12** months.

1

The Guinea Pig Club had initially created a blazer badge in a circular form.

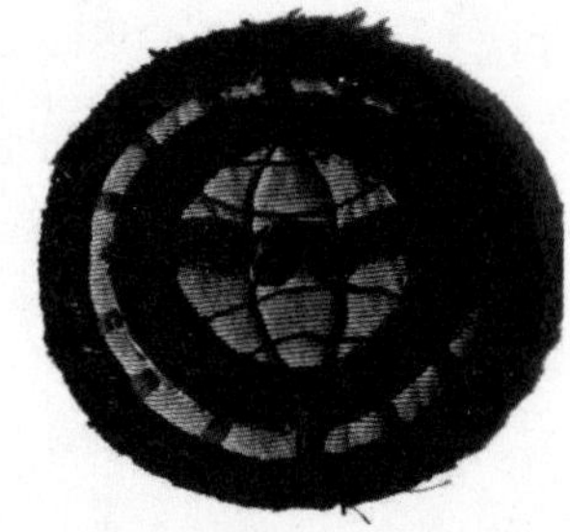

The early-design woven Guinea Pig Club blazer badge.

220

Sir Archibald McIndoe addressed this number of Guinea Pigs present at the 1948 annual dinner with the sobering thought that combined, they shared some **2,000** operations and they had lost and regained enough skin to paper the walls of the room where they sat.[18]

649

It was accepted that the Guinea Pig Club had this many members when Ward Three closed in 1948. Archibald McIndoe and his team would have treated thousands of burns victims, including civilians and patients from the other military services. Amongst them, the tank commander and future Conservative member of Parliament, Robert Boscawen. McIndoe even reached out to Allied prisoner of war camp hospitals. By example, the hospital at Stalag IXB Bad Soden was managed by Major David Charters. He was an eye specialist before the war and cared for Flying Officer Maurice Buttler a Coastal Command navigator, who was captured after his Hudson was shot down on 10 February 1943. Maurice had burns to his hands and face and spent months in a Luftwaffe hospital before arriving at Stalag IXB. Major Charters wrote to McIndoe to seek advice. Using improvised instruments and Red Cross supplies, Charters treated Buttler for **8** months before he was repatriated in 1944 and referred to McIndoe at East Grinstead.[19] Major David Charters was also the individual who assisted the previously mentioned Russian prisoner of war Guinea Pig, Vladimir Razumov.

1948

On 5 July that year the Queen Victoria Hospital, passed into Governmental control as part of the new National Health Service which resulted in the Hospital Management Committee no longer having control of the affairs of the hospital.

600

Archibald McIndoe undertook a **3**-month lecture tour in the United States and Canada in 1948. *Time* magazine published an article in September of that year titled 'The man who makes faces'.[20] McIndoe referenced his **600** cases undertaken at the Queen Victoria Hospital in the article and it was a figure he never deviated from in any of his lectures.

150

The immediate post-war Guinea Pig Club reunions, initially called Guinea Pig Lost Weekends, were attended on average by this number of Guinea Pigs. Members often travelled to East Grinstead on the Friday. Saturday mornings had an open invitation to meet and review medical situations with Archibald McIndoe. Lunchtime was normally a pub event, with darts whilst the evening was an organised dinner. These arrangements changed and evolved as the years progressed. Efforts inevitably took place to have a celebrity, a star of screen stage or music to appear. The 1949 dinner reunion at the Whitehall saw three mechanical horses known as 'Mobo Broncos' which were ridden by Johnny Maguire, an entertaining personality of that time. Inevitably, it developed into a competitive horse race for Guinea Pigs across the dance floor.

1

Only one Guinea Pig Club member took part in flying food and supplies into post-war western Germany. William Simpson flew privately for the Lancashire Aircraft Corporation whose aircraft was chartered to engage in the Berlin Airlift supply flights which took place between June 1948 to May 1949. By providing a monumental number of flights into Germany the Soviet Union's actions which had intentionally blocked the Western Allies' railway, road, and canal access to the sectors of Berlin under Western control were broken. In addition to military flights, there were over **13,000** civil aircraft flights undertaken by **35** civil four engine aircraft during the Berlin Airlift. The cost to the British taxpayers was estimated at approximately **£8,600,000**.[21]

6

The number of South African Guinea Pigs who met with Archibald McIndoe during his visits to their home country. Those he is known to have met were Godfrey Edmonds, Bill Bourne, Graham Lawson, Barney Levin, Noel Berrington-Pickett and Bruce Loneon. The latter had the distinction of joining the club with a sporting facial fracture injury in 1943.[22] McIndoe had worked to establish the African Medical and Research Foundation, his vision was for lasting health change in Africa.

1st

The first occasion whereby high-ranking military dignitaries were absent from the top table at the annual dinner occurred on 3 September 1949. Founder members of the Guinea Pig Club that were able to attend, continued to be seated with Sir Archibald McIndoe on the top table.

100

The approximate number of Guinea Pigs who attended the 1949 annual dinner.

1,000

The minimum order of proposed Guinea Pig Club ties that was required to be ordered from the manufacturers in 1949. At a cost of **£600**, it was regarded as too expensive to proceed. However, the concept of delivering a club tie remained on the agenda.

8

Guinea Pig Hugh Parratt returned to the Queen Victoria Hospital for an additional operation to his foot. Hugh was a Wireless Operator who had previously been awarded the Distinguished Flying Medal. He probably lost the heel portion of his foot when his bomber crashed into a marshalling yard from **20,000ft** in a flat spin over Germany in December 1944. Hugh arrived at East Grinstead hospital on 23 October 1945 where **8** operations relating to his prior injuries were undertaken.[23]

5/-

5 shillings, the equivalent of 50p in decimal currency, were charged for each Guinea Pig Club member wearing their badges on entrance to the Eve-of-Dinner dance at the Rainbow Ballroom, Whitehall in September 1950. An additional **2** shillings and **6** pence was charged should no badge be worn.

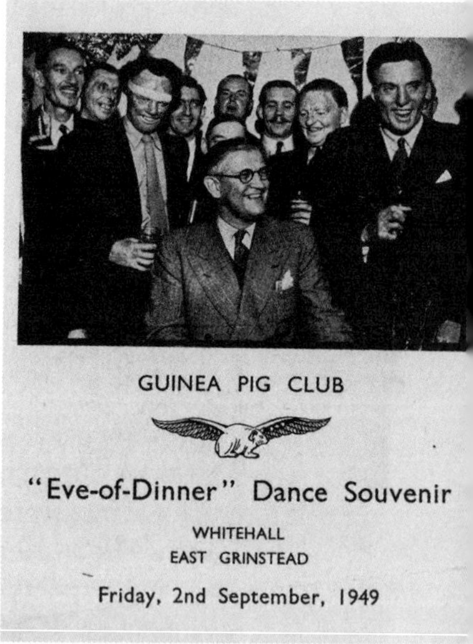

1949 Guinea Pig Club eve-of-dinner dance invitation at the Whitehall.

2nd

A stolen and abandoned lorry on an unlit main road in 1950 resulted in a collision which was impossible to have been avoided for Guinea Pig Thomas Voges. The accident knocked him unconscious with head injuries, a badly-damaged eye and smashed hand. After initial medical treatment, Thomas was taken to the Queen Victoria Hospital. It was his **2nd** admission into the East Grinstead hospital as Thomas' Wellington bomber had crashed in training on 3 May 1942. He had **3** operations to repair the burn injuries to his face neck and hands. It is unknown how many additional operations were undertaken after the road accident.[24]

8/6

The first Guinea Pig Club tie became available for members to purchase at a cost of **8** shillings and **6** pence in December 1950. Clothing coupons which had controlled rationing were still present but officially ceased in 1951.[25]

155

The Whitehall renovations in 1950 saw the Club's annual dinner relocate to the Felbridge Hotel near East Grinstead. The annual event was now well known as 'The Lost Weekend'. **155** Guinea Pigs attended that year's event.

1

Donald Robert Gordon Attwater received medical training at Halton and Rauceby Hospital. He met Archibald McIndoe and started nursing at Queen Victoria Hospital on 1 January 1952. Additionally, he was ordained as a reverend in November 1961 and became Senior Nursing Officer in 1971. In addition to being a nursing professional and an Evangelical Reverend, he helped many of the Guinea Pigs throughout their ongoing treatments. Tea or dinner invitations were frequently undertaken for them at his family home in Smallfield, Surrey. Donald Attwater was always present whenever possible at the annual reunions. As the Guinea Pig Club's honorary chaplain, he would say grace at the formal dinners. He retired from the Queen Victoria Hospital in 1989.[26]

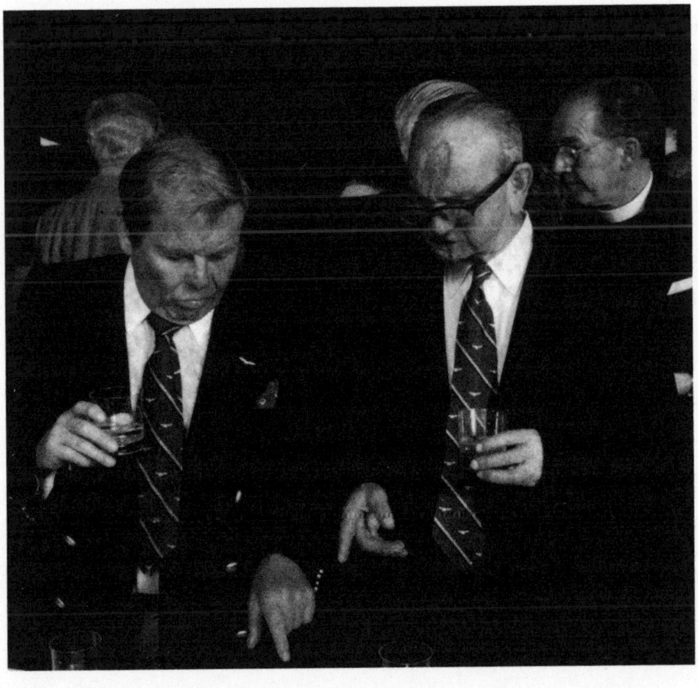

Guinea Pig Tubby Taylor on the left alongside another Guinea Pig Reverend Donald Attwater, the club's honorary chaplain, standing far right. (*Image via Steve Attwater*)

1951 Jimmy Edwards, so often wrongly regarded as a Guinea Pig himself, entertained at the club reunion on 26 October of that year, then again on 24 October 1952 and by popular request he appeared once more on 23 October 1953. In 1940 he volunteered for the Royal Air Force and trained to become a pilot. He was shot down and suffered burns when his Dakota suffered an engine fire whilst making a third pass over Arnhem in September 1944. Jimmy Edwards received an immediate Distinguished Flying Cross for his gallantry. No doubt this explains the connectivity between the Guinea Pig Club and the boldly-moustached humourist and entertainer who chose to wear his splendid facial hair to hide his burn scarring.[27]

1953 Archibald McIndoe told Guinea Pigs gathered at East Grinstead for the annual reunion that year: 'I am filled with amazement and deep respect at the way in which practically all of you have become men in your own right, standing on your own feet and facing the world fearlessly. Such are the truly satisfying results of our organization, our Guinea Pig Club.'

1955 Max Bygraves entertained the Guinea Pigs on 28 October that year. He returned to perform on other reunions alongside other highly-rated entertainers of that time.

1957 The original newsletter front cover artwork ceased illustrating the two prominently bandaged Guinea Pigs in that year. Reduced in size, they were seen alongside what were to be differing images of personalities of the time.

1 Sir Archibald McIndoe purchased Caxton Manor, Wall Hill, Forest Row in the mid-1950s. Caxton Manor was an impressive picturesque timber-framed house dating back to the fifteenth century, set within a five-acre garden.

150 The number of Guinea Pigs that attended the **15th** annual reunion in 1956.

0 It is unknown where the flamboyant Guinea Pig Dennis Taylor acquired his toilet pan-shaped drinking jug from. The jug became his symbol of frivolity and features in many images taken at numerous events. The club newsletter booklet featured a full-page illustration of his jug.[28] Known as 'Tubby' Taylor, he also became renowned for inevitably jumping fully clad into the Felbridge Hotel swimming pool at the reunions. That dunking may well be connected to his membership of the Goldfish Club.

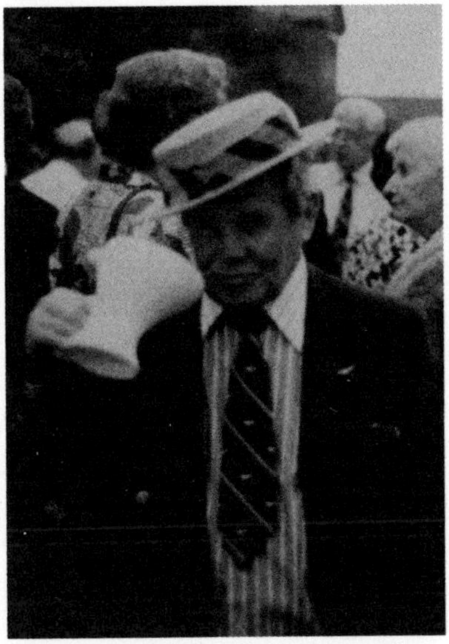

'Tubby' Taylor wearing the Guinea Pig Club tie and holding his toilet pan beer mug which was inevitably seen at every latter annual reunion.

1957 The Guinea Pig public house, named in honour of the club was officially opened in that year and was situated close to the East Grinstead Hospital in Holtye Avenue. The pub predictably became a favourite with veterans and patients alike. Last orders were called for the final time in 2008, when it closed its doors. The closure was to make way for a housing development. The pub was demolished in 2009 but the name lives on at the site through the development being called Guinea Pig Place.

1 The original pub sign is now an exhibit in the East Grinstead Museum.

1 Josef Kapka was a remarkable Guinea Pig who 'escaped' from behind the Iron Curtain to attend a reunion. His presence at Ye Olde Felbridge hotel in 1957 was published in the press: 'As usual there were a number of unexpected members who turned up for the re-union dinner at Ye Olde Felbridge hotel, and distinguished among them was a former Czech pilot, Josef Kapka, who has escaped from behind the Iron Curtain. For seven years he had been in a Communist Concentration Camp. He has now rejoined his English wife, a wartime W.A.A.F .... It was just ten years since he last attended a Guinea Pig re-union. He is now to be looked after by the Guinea Pig Club while he and his wife are settling down. They will find him a job, helping him, as they have done for so many, to start life afresh.'[29]

10 Sir Archibald McIndoe wrote a 'Foreword' in the book written by Czechoslovakian Guinea Pig Jo Capka. McIndoe wrote: 'He was eventually shot down by the rear gunner of what appeared to be a damaged American Liberator but which was in fact a German decoy. In this engagement he was severely injured in the face and came under my care.' McIndoe had selected him for his care when he undertook a visit to the hospital at Ely. It was there that Capka's eye had been removed. McIndoe subsequently operated upon Jo Capka in October 1944. He suffered burns to his forehead and arms in addition to the facial wounds. Squadron Leader Moore then operated upon his skin grafts in February 1945 and released scaring on his elbow in January 1946. Jo Capka returned to Czechoslovakia but was later arrested by the ruling Communist regime. They sentenced him to **10** years hard labour, the first year of which was in solitary confinement. He was released in 1957, whereby he returned to England. His book, *Red Sky at Night*, was published in 1958. The brave Capka had received the British Distinguished Flying Medal and the French Croix de Guerre to accompany his home countries service awards.

6

The number of positions of 'Honorary Guinea Pig' permitted. Lord Portal, Lord Tedder, Sir John Slessor and Sir John Cordingley occupied **4** positions. **2** vacancies were consistently carried without occupancy.[30] Sir Victor Sassoon and Clifford Stone were both appointed 'Honorary Guinea Pigs' to fill naturally occurring vacancies. Another known 'Honorary Guinea Pig' was Doctor Tom Cochrane, a plastic surgeon who had supported the Guinea Pigs in many ways, giving his time selflessly with advice on medical, social and pension problems.[31]

100

Battle of Britain Guinea Pig, Maurice Mounsdon had his centenarian milestone marked by a dedicated flypast to him by the RAF Red Arrows display team.

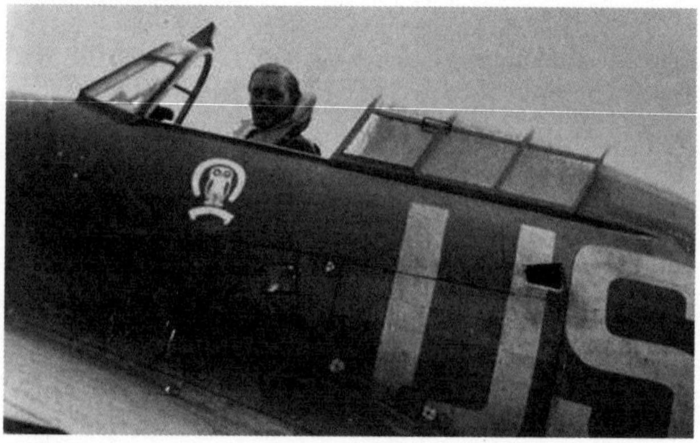

Maurice Mounsdon in the cockpit of his 56 Squadron Hurricane in 1940. The owl and horseshoe emblem under which a banner with the inscription 'Oiseau de Morte' – translated as 'Bird of Death'.

1958

In that year, Sir Archibald McIndoe appeared on the BBC's *The Week's Good Cause* programme to appeal for financial support. In speaking of the sacrifices made by members of the RAF, he said: 'How can we right the balance of payment. We can't do it personally the job is too big, but the Royal Air Force Benevolent Fund will do it for us, if you will help.' The appeal raised £5,000.

1958

The Freedom of the City of London was awarded to 'Sir Archibald Hector McIndoe, Kt. C.B.E. Citizen of London' in the Mayoral period of 'Sir Denis Henry Truscott, Kt., T.D.' on 19 March that year.

20,000

Also in 1958, Sir Archibald McIndoe in his Bradshaw lecture pronounced that more than **20,000** men in the RAF had been 'incinerated with or without injuries'. Clearly Sir Archibald was referencing the loss of life in fires within aircraft across many scenarios and that **4,500** burned aircrew were recovered from crashed planes or parachuted in flames to safety, not forgetting ground staff who had suffered from burns as a result of explosions and fires. **3,600** sustained injuries on the face and hands, and practically all of these were treated in Royal Air Force Burns Units under centralised control. Of these men **600** in England, and others later from the Middle East, were transferred to East Grinstead, of which **200** were regarded as of major severity or as total facial burns.[32]

£10,000

During the later war years, Archibald McIndoe and Neville Blond at Gotwick Manor, Hammerwood began formulating the idea for an independent research centre. Neville Blond was serving as a British trade adviser at the time when increased demands were being made on the Ministry of Health following the expansion of the National Health Service. In 1958 government funding was inevitably not going to be available. Mr and Mrs Blond generously provided the sum of £10,000 to construct the research building at their expense. The Blond McIndoe Centre for Medical Research at East Grinstead Hospital opened in 1960. It has become a world-renowned medical research institute pioneering treatments for burn injuries. Elaine and Neville Blond were the founding patrons and principal fundraisers for the centre. The couple also funded research fellowships and treatment centres at the Queen Victoria Hospital, East Grinstead. Neville died in 1970 and Elaine died in 1985.

1

At least **1** Guinea Pig appeared in film in the years after the war. Bill Foxley made an appearance in 1969. His role in the film *Battle of Britain* gave significant awareness of the facial burns suffered by the early burn casualties of that time. However, he was actually a casualty from within a Wellington bomber who sustained his burns in attempting to rescue a crewmate following a crash during training.

5

At least this number of Guinea Pigs appeared on the long-running biographical television documentary *This is Your Life* and presented with the 'Big Red Book'. One of these men was the remarkable Colin Hodgkinson, who appeared in the episode that was broadcast live on 7 October 1957. Bill Simpson, Geoffrey Page, Tom Gleave and Joe Capka were the other participants. The recipient's life story was presented to them in the form of an impressive red-bound book.

2

An anonymous well-wisher donated **2** return air tickets for two overseas Guinea Pigs to attend the 1951 annual meeting. A draw concluded that an Australian and a South African club member would benefit from the generous gift.[33]

49

Theatre sister Jill Mullins, a key member of McIndoe's team in the operating theatres and a vital member of the original three at East Grinstead, remained as McIndoe's preferred surgical assistant until 1957. She moved to South Africa with her husband's business but tragically died of a stroke whilst travelling to Johannesburg in 1959, aged just **49**. Sir McIndoe was devastated by her death and praised her many remarkable qualities in a touching tribute in the Guinea Pig magazine. He wrote: 'Sometimes I had to operate without her, to me it was hell.'[34] Little doubt exists that Mullins and McIndoe had a very close relationship bounded by professional respect in equal measures.

5

On 16 October 1959, the governments of the United Kingdom and the Federal Republic of Germany made an agreement about the future care of the remains of German military personnel who at that time were interred in various local cemeteries. It was agreed that the remains would be transferred to a single central cemetery established on Cannock Chase in Staffordshire. This applied to the Luftwaffe casualties over East Grinstead and in the Queen Victoria Hospital. They were Hermann Winkelmann, Rudolf Precht, Hubert Kasing, Walter Domenig and Hans Strahlendorf. These **5** Luftwaffe airmen were reinterred at Cannock Chase cemetery.[35]

1960 Sir Archibald McIndoe died in his sleep in London on 11 April that year. He was **59** years of age.

1st The first annual dinner without Sir Archibald McIndoe took place on 24 September 1960.

1961 A unique event involved the horse 'St. Paddy' owned by Sir Victor Sassoon, the honorary Guinea Pig club member and benefactor to the club and hospital. The horse won the Eclipse Stake race in that year whilst it carried Sir Sassoon's Guinea Pig Badge. As a celebration one stud fee per year from his stables was thereafter donated to the Guinea Pig Club's funds.[36] Sir Victor had served in the Royal Flying Corps in the First World War. He survived a plane crash in 1916 in which he sustained leg injuries that plagued him for the rest of his life. He often attended annual club reunions in a wheelchair.

14 The London residence of Archibald McIndoe was Flat **14**, Avenue Court, Chelsea. That property now displays an English Heritage Blue Plaque of Honour in recognition of his contribution to society.

71 An English Heritage plaque resides on the wall of Sir Harold Gillies' London residence at **71** Frognall, Hampstead, Camden which sits within proximity to Hampstead Village. It records the fact that he was a pioneer plastic surgeon. He died on 10 September 1960.

1 Prince Philip, the Duke of Edinburgh, became resident president for the remainder of the Guinea Pig Club's existence.

3 The number of silver Guinea Pig Club brooches commissioned to be presented on 23 September 1961 to Lady McIndoe, and her daughters Adonia and Venora.[37]

1 Lady McIndoe presented the Royal Air Force Church St Clement Danes in London with an altar chair carved with the Guinea Pig Wings and dedicated to Sir McIndoe. Known as an Episcopal seat, the seat cushion carries the insignia of the four Orders of Chivalry awarded to McIndoe: the Polish Order of St Stanislas, the Czech Order of the White Lion, the French Legion of Honour, and the Dutch Order of Orange-Nassau. The church holds the Books of Remembrance to all those who have died in service in the RAF. Kneelers also record the lives of pilots, and airmen and others lost during the Second

World War. Each memorial kneeler carries the initials of a person lost and was stitched by hand. On the night of 10 May 1941, St. Clement Danes was struck by direct hits from incendiary bombs and shrapnel. As a result of the German bombing, the church was completely destroyed with only the **4** walls and spire remaining standing. Following an appeal for funds the painstaking rebuilding work of recreating the important structure to the original design took place. In 1958, St. Clement Danes was consecrated as the Central Church of the Royal Air Force and opened by Her Majesty Queen Elizabeth II. High above the altar is an ornately carved coat of arms of Queen Elizabeth II. The Latin inscription below the crest translates as 'Built by Christopher Wren 1681. Destroyed by the thunderbolts of air warfare 1941. Restored by the Royal Air Force 1958.' Sir Archibald McIndoe's legacy is very much evidenced by the fact that following his death in April 1960 and to this day, he is the only civilian to have his ashes interred within the church.

1963

On 6 July that year, Lady Connie McIndoe married Clifford Sabey.[38] The Guinea Pig Club presented a solid silver Guinea Pig for their wedding gift. It was cast replicating a large-scale membership badge complete with wings.

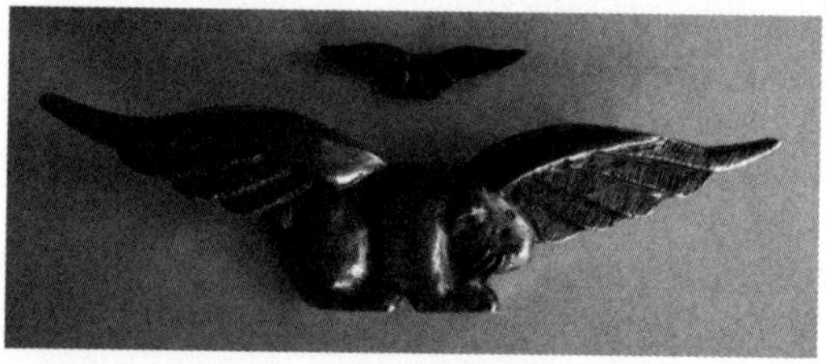

An example of the club's 1991 anniversary badge is seen with a presentation solid silver large-scale membership badge. The anniversary badges were commissioned by the Guinea Pig Club and cast by Klondyke Jewellers Limited. The master jeweller responsible was John Balcombe Meaden of Haywards Health, Sussex. Both items carry the maker's identity of KJ Ltd. This large-scale Guinea Pig Club badge is a unique example which was retained after casting by Mrs Sally Meaden.

35/-

35 shillings, the cost to purchase a Guinea Pig Club wall plaque which had been commissioned and made available to the club members.[39]

1964

The highly popular singer Cilla Black entertained at the Guinea Pig Club reunion on 25 September that year.

1966 Dick Emery, who in the 1960s and 1970s became one of the most successful comics on television, entertained the Guinea Pigs on 23 September that year. He was followed by Arthur Askey, Joe Brown and Mike Yarwood into the 1970s. Tommy Trinder and Reg Varney with Leslie Crowther entertained into the 1980s. The Guinea Pig Club could not have been better recognised by more significant entertainers of those times.

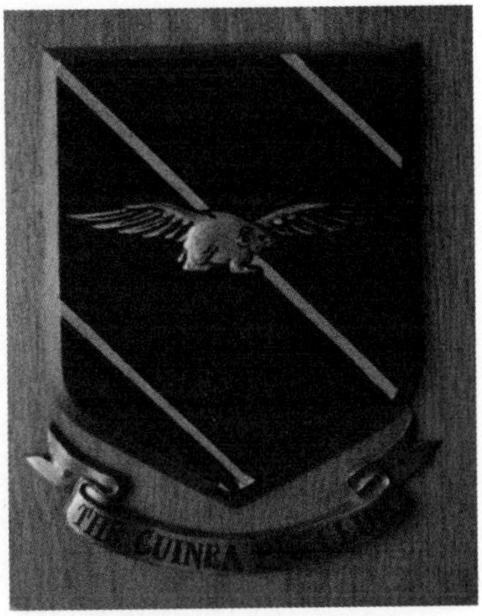

The wooden wall plaque with embossed relief Guinea Pig was presented to dignitaries and contributors in acknowledging support of the club. St Swithun's Church, in Church Lane, East Grinstead has a plaque on display. There are also memorials on the wall honouring some of those killed in the Whitehall Bombing on 9 July 1943, and the three killed by the flying bomb on 12 July 1944. Several Guinea Pig weddings took place in this church. The church's fifth clerestory window, has the Guinea Pig club's badge design set within the decorative glass which surrounds the central picture. These were inset in the installations during the late 1980s.

18 The number of Canadian Guinea Pigs who crossed the Atlantic along with Ross Tilley to attend the 1971 reunion. Group Captain Douglas Bader was an invited guest on what was the **30th** anniversary of the founding of the club.

39 The **39th** annual club dinner took place in 1980 with a full-size replica Spitfire displayed on the forecourt at the Felbridge Hotel.

865 The Battle of Britain Spitfire pilot Jack Mann is the only member of the Guinea Pig Club to have been kidnapped and held hostage. He had been shot down **6** times and awarded the Distinguished Flying Medal in April 1941. 'This airman has displayed great keenness in his many operations against the enemy and has destroyed at least four of their aircraft. His enthusiasm and fighting spirit have been outstanding and this was particularly displayed on one occasion when, during a patrol, his aircraft was severely damaged through enemy action. With great presence of mind, and despite his aircraft being uncontrollable at the time, he warned his flight commander by radio telephone of the danger from a rear attack by enemy aircraft and almost certainly saved the commander from being shot down.'[40] He was wounded multiple times during his operational flying becoming a member of the Guinea Pig Club with burns and gunshot injuries on 4 April 1941. In retirement in Beirut in 1989, the Revolutionary Justice Organisation took him prisoner on 12 May. Jack Mann, always known as Jackie spent his entire captivity in solitary confinement. He was not released until 24 September 1991 at the age of **77**. He had spent **865** days in captivity. He was brought back to Britain, given a fly-past by Spitfires and returned into the arms of his wife. He underwent recuperation at the Air Force station Lyneham before moving to Cyprus. Jack Mann was made a Commander of the Order of the British Empire in the New Year Honours list of 1992 'For courage and fortitude while held hostage in the Lebanon'. He died at his home in Nicosia aged **81**.

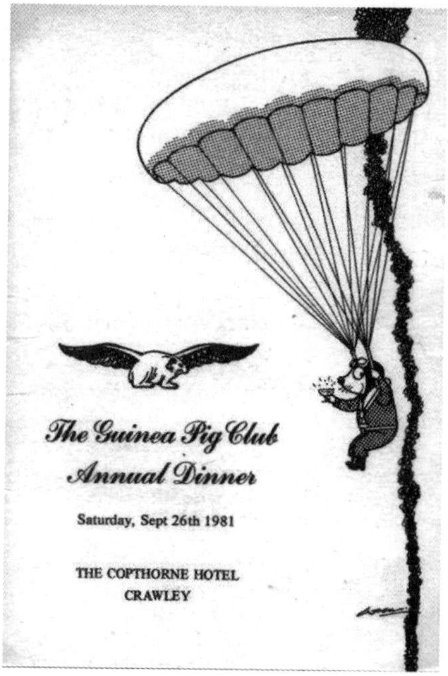

The menu card for the Guinea Pig Club annual reunion dinner on 26 September 1981.

1 Members of the Guinea Pig Club together with their partners visited the Rutherford Appleton Laboratory at Didcot in Oxfordshire on 5 June 1982. The Laboratory presented the Chief Guinea Pig Tom Gleave with a commemorative plate made at the laboratory. The

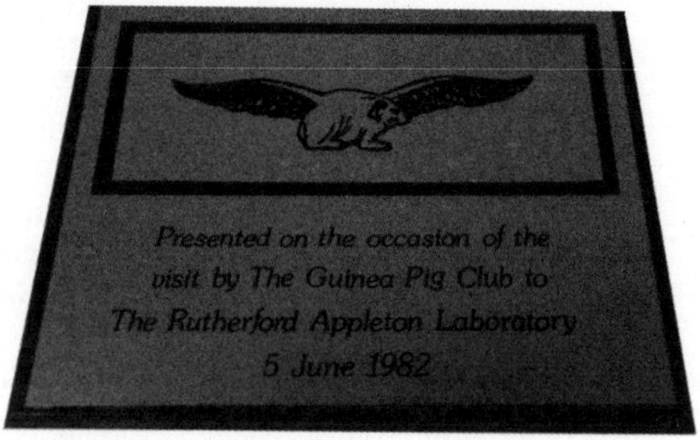
Presented on the occasion of the
visit by The Guinea Pig Club to
The Rutherford Appleton Laboratory
5 June 1982

A plaque presented to the Guinea Pig Club commemorating the official visit to the Rutherford Appleton Laboratory on 5 June 1982.

group toured both the laser Bio Medical unit and the Electron beam millimetre-wave telescope facilities.

1 **1** Spitfire, Serial Number AB910 of the Battle of Britain Memorial Flight, carried the Guinea Pig Club badge prominently painted on its nose cowling in the 1990 flying season.

50 In 1991, the Felbridge Hotel in East Grinstead hosted the club's **50th** anniversary reunion. The club commissioned engraved numbered gold gilt Guinea Pig Club membership badges to celebrate the occasion. The President, Prince Philip was in attendance. The author met several club members at this event.

50 In August 1994 at Victoria, the capital of British Columbia, Canada, the **50th** anniversary reunion of the 'Canadian Wing' of the Guinea Pig Club was celebrated. The attendees each received an engraved glass recognising the event.

643 In the millennium year of 2000, a sign writer was commissioned to create a Roll of Honour naming the **643** members of the Guinea Pig Club. This impressive wooden panel was officially unveiled at the East Grinstead Hospital on 5 November 2003.

50 A proposal was made at the Guinea Pig Club's annual meeting in 2001 that when there were only **50** members left in the club, it should be wound up. This proposal was voted down by those present, it being said that as long as there were **2** members who could raise a glass to each other, then the club should continue and this is exactly what happened.

2004 Henry Standen's Guinea Pig artwork finally disappeared entirely from the front cover of the club's newsletters in that year. Those 21st-century publications were more commonly referred to as magazines.

120 By 2004, there were just **120** Guinea Pig Club members remaining, **34** of whom were Canadian.

44 The final edition of the club newsletter in 2004 was printed with this many pages of content by Metloc's printers at Loughton Essex. The final article published by the club was about the Queen Victoria Blond McIndoe Research Foundation.

97

The number of Guinea Pigs registered with the club in 2007 was **97** with **57** resident in Britain and **40** elsewhere in the world.

66

The Club's last ever-annual dinner saw that many members in attendance. This took place on Saturday, 13 October 2007, in the presence of Prince Philip. At the time of the dinner, the youngest member was aged **82** and the oldest was **102**.

7ft

A statue commemorating McIndoe's work was unveiled by The Princess Royal in front of Sackville College, at the junction of College Lane and East Grinstead's historic High Street, in June 2014. Commissioned by the Blond McIndoe Research Foundation, a fundraising target of £175,000 was reached with considerable support from McIndoe's family. The 7ft tall statue, which depicts the surgeon with a convalescing serviceman was the work of sculptor Martin Jennings. In front of the statue is the following inscription: 'He led a pioneering team whose treatment gave the lives back to

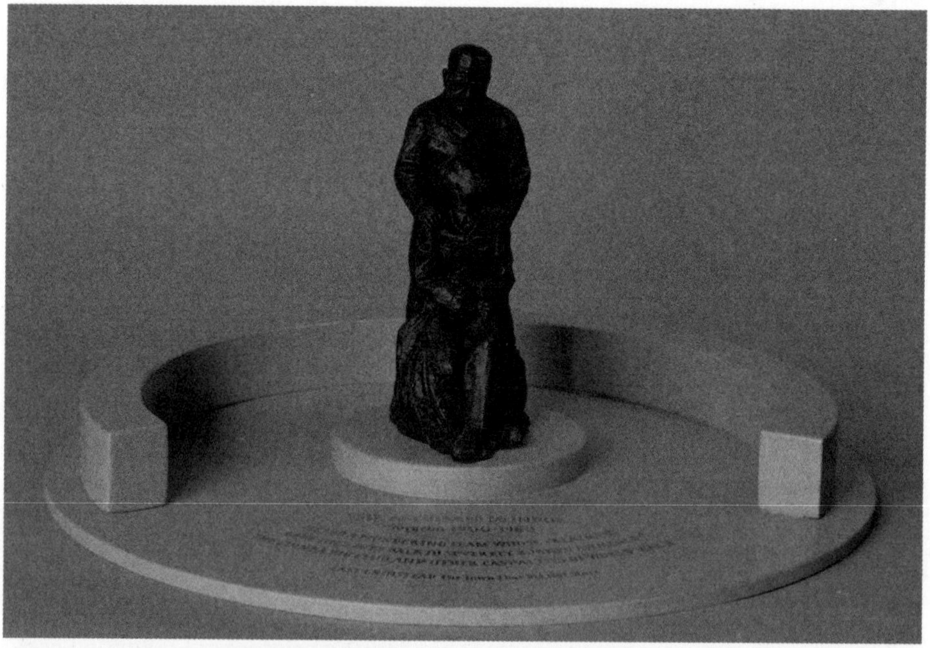

The sculptor Martin Jennings' design model for the bronze statue of Sir Archibald McIndoe. With a patient, the bronze is set within a round plinth with carved script detail. The sculptor's father Michael Jennings, had been wounded in a tank battle in Holland in 1944. He was treated at the Queen Victoria Hospital by McIndoe's colleague Percy Jayes. The sculptor's model can be seen on display at the East Grinstead Museum.

severely burned airmen of the Guinea Pig Club and other casualties of World War II.'

17

There were believed to be just **17** surviving Guinea Pigs in the world on the eve of 2017.

0

Prince Philip, the Duke of Edinburgh, the sitting president of the Guinea Pig Club, died on 9 April 2021.

101

The Guinea Pig Club ceased functioning after the last two members, Sam Gallop and Jan Black, both passed away in November 2023. They died within **10** days of each other, both aged **101**. Bob Marchant, the club's secretary, finally closed the records of the Guinea Pig Club.

1

There is a single stained glass window that incorporates the logo of the Guinea Pig Club. This is in St Swithun's Church, East Grinstead. The church had close links with the Guinea Pigs, an annual service was always held during the reunion weekend. In the church there is a memorial tablet dedicated to Henry Standen, and his fellow Guinea Pigs. While in the small chapel, to the left of the main altar there is a chair in memory of Chief Guinea Pig, Group Captain Tom Gleave.

11

The number of streets and roads in East Grinstead that have been named in honour of the Club. These names are notably found on the estate opposite the hospital in Holtye Road. Burns Way, Wagg Close, Stirling Way, Wellington Gate, Gleave Close, Merlin Way, Kindersley Close, Hillary Close, Spitfire Court, Blenheim Close and McIndoe Road.

1

The original Allen & Hanbury operating table which Archibald McIndoe used throughout the Second World War was salvaged and preserved by Bob

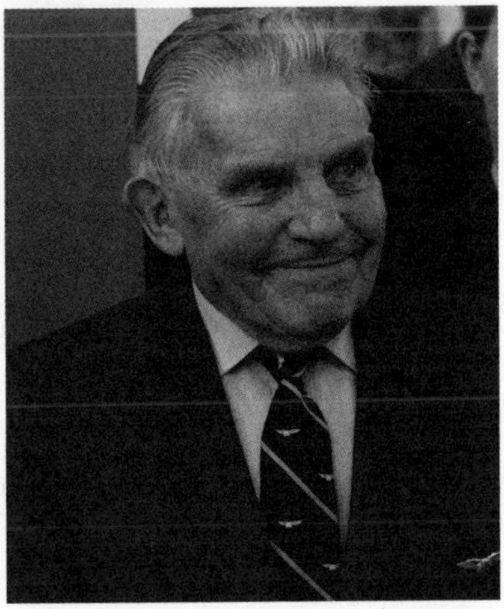

The late Bob Marchant who worked alongside Archibald McIndoe and was the final Guinea Pig Club membership secretary. A trustee of the East Grinstead Museum who willingly gave the author much time over many years with the research into the Guinea Pig Club. Bob Marchant seen wearing his honorary club tie and club membership badge. (*Image via Ian Marchant*)

Marchant. That operating table is now an exhibit and on display at the East Grinstead Museum.

2m

The Guinea Pig Club memorial, located at the National Memorial Arboretum in Alrewas, Staffordshire stands at **2** meters tall. It was unveiled by the Duke of Edinburgh on 2 November 2016. The spiralling vapour trail from the plane forms the outline of the face of Sir Archibald MacIndoe. The right-hand side edge is polished and smooth and shaped like a Spitfire wing. As well as the Club emblem, the memorial also carries an inscription provided by the Guinea Pig, Sandy Saunders. 'Out of the flames came inspiration.'

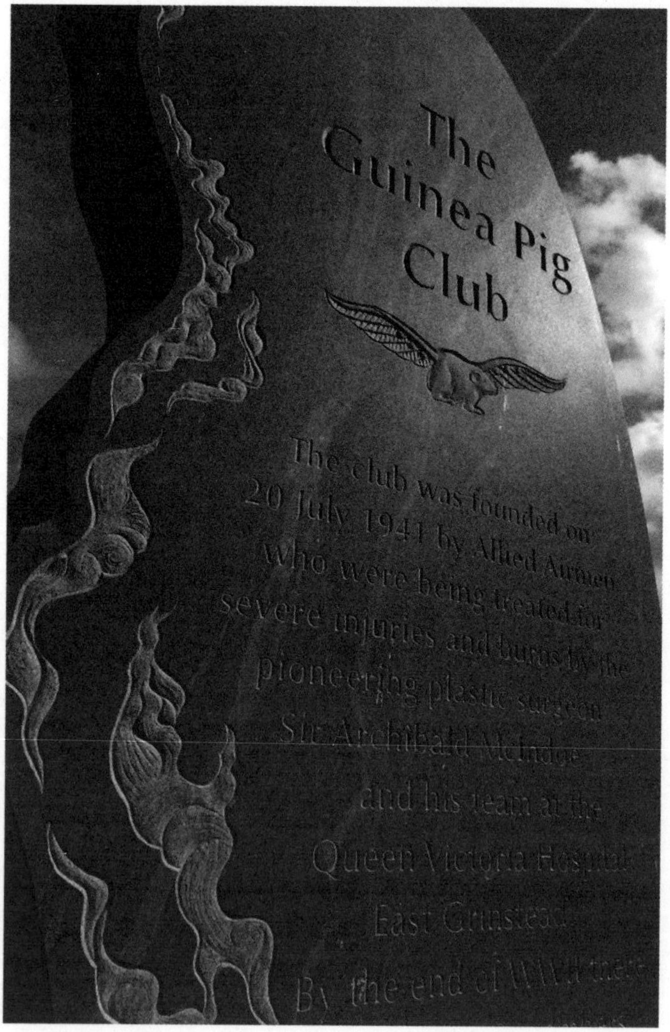
The Guinea Pig Club
The club was founded on
20 July 1941 by Allied Airmen
who were being treated for
and his team at the
East Grinstead

The National Memorial Arboretum Guinea Pig Club memorial carved from green Cumbrian slate by artist Graeme Mitcheson. The design features a crashed Hurricane at the bottom of the memorial with smoke trail weaving down from the top. The green slate naturally exposed these distinctive white streaks towards the bottom of the stone which coincidentally provided the flames of the burning Hurricane aircraft. The text is carved into the smooth surface and the logo of the Guinea Pig Club is carved at the top of the memorial.

Conclusion

Probably no better understanding of the impact upon the men Archibald McIndoe treated could be better described than by the wife of the valiant Czechoslovakian Guinea Pig Josef Koukal. His wife was with him when he passed away on 23 February 1980, aged 68. His wife watched Josef as he stood in front of the framed photograph of Sir Archibald McIndoe. Josef looked at the man who had operated upon him endless times over a two-year period. He studied the photograph for about a minute, and then Josef suddenly collapsed and died.[1]

No longer will the Guinea Pig Club's anthem echo anywhere in the world. Those who composed the words and the men who sung them with pride are no more.

The Roll of Honour of the men who were treated at the Queen Victoria Hospital is displayed in the corridor of the Canadian Wing at Queen Victoria Hospital. There are 15 columns holding **643** names painted in gold beneath the emblem of the Guinea Pig.

<u>NAMES PRESENT ON MEMORIAL BOARD BUT MISSING FROM THE 1963 PUBLISHED LIST.</u>

J.G. ADAMS. C.G.D. BUTLER. R.G. CHITHAM. M. COOTE. F. COPPOCK. D. DAVEY. G. EDMUNDS [SAAF] G. EDMONSTON. R. HILLARY. J.K. KELLY. E.S. LOCK. A. NESBITT. L.J. SOMERS. B. OWEN-SMITH. J.W. SQUIER. R. TATAJCZAK.

<u>NAMES MISSING FROM BOTH MEMORIAL BOARD AND 1963 PUBLISHED LIST.</u>

B. OWEN-SMITH. F.H. MAHN. J.P. CALDER. G. SHAUGHNESSY. H. AVERY.[2]

<u>NAME MISSING ON MEMORIAL BOARD BUT PRESENT IN 1963 PUBLISHED LIST.</u>

H. ANDERSON [3]

<u>NAMES ON MEMORIAL BOARD UNABLE TO BE IDENTIFIED</u>

P. A. S. WOODWARK. G. BUTCHER. J. K. KELLY. D. HARVY. R. TATAJCZAK. H. CURWAIN. R. WHAM.

Notes

Chapter 1: The Founding of Friendships Amongst Guinea Pig Patients

1. AIR 81/1610 Aircraftman W. Cruickshank injured; Pilot Officer G. Frain, Pilot Officer C. Watt, Aircraftman L. Steele: uninjured. Anson N5274, 612 Squadron; aircraft accident, 28 October 1939.
2. *The Royal Air Force Medical Services* Volume 1 'Administration' by Squadron Leader S. C. Rexford-Welch, p. 301.
3. Ward Three was the dedicated burns ward in the hospital.
4. 'Who's Who in the Guinea Pig Club', *The Guinea Pig*, August 1952.
5. Bob Marchant, Guinea Pig Club secretary.
6. AIR 81 – Air Ministry: P4 (Cas) Files relating to casualties suffered during air operations and aircraft accidents 1939-1945.
7. Kenneth Wynn, *Men of the Battle of Britain* (Gliddon Books, 1989).
8. Ibid. The rule also required at least two operations to have been undertaken which appears never to have been upheld.
9. Pre-decimalisation figure shown. On 15 February 1971 one shilling 1/- became 5p
10. 'Guinea Pigs and Friends on Parade', *The Guinea Pig*, Summer 1962, p. 13.
11. East Grinstead Museum data confirms Robert Smith-Barry's age of 54.
12. Deed poll 15 December 1949, and the Supreme Court of Judicature on 29 December 1949, DEREK DUDLEY MARTIN, of 135 Heene Road, Worthing, Sussex, citizen of the United Kingdom and Colonies by birth, renounced and abandoned the names of Dudley Martin Butcher and Derek Dudley Martin Butcher. Dated 2 day of January, 1950.
13. Example – National Archives AIR78 records reveals 109 men with the registration name Dewar.
14. Kenneth Wynn, *Men of the Battle of Britain* (Gliddon Books, 1989).
15. BAPRAS author's communications, The British Association of Plastic, Reconstructive and Aesthetic Surgeons.
16. Rexford Welch casualty and medical statistics of WWII, p. 460.
17. Ibid.
18. *The Guinea Pig*, New Year 1991, p. 10.
19. Kenneth Wynn, *Men of the Battle of Britain* (Gliddon Books, 1989).
20. Annual dinner speech, 2 September 1950
21. Bob Marchant, Guinea Pig Club membership secretary.
22. Statistics for known nationalities and trades in service originates from Bob Marchant and the East Grinstead Museum data.
23. Dr Jenkins was a qualified anaesthetist who also worked at Queen Victoria Hospital theatre during his rehabilitation in 1946.
24. Dr Robert G. Chitham, *The Guinea Pig*, New Year 1994, pp. 5–6.
25. Rita Donovan, 'As for the Canadians', *The Guinea Pig*, New Year 1994, p. 13. Note that the Canadian statistics are conflicting across several sources.

26. AIR 81/11039 Pilot Officer F. H. W. Keene from Argentina volunteered to fly with the RAF. His aircraft was hit by enemy anti-aircraft fire west of Tripoli, Libya. Prisoners of war with burns. Hospital ship to England. East Grinstead Hospital late 1944.
27. RCAF J4695 R.O.4. records and newspaper cutting.
28. James J. Halley, *Royal Air Force Aircraft L1000-N9999* (Air Britain, 1983). *Flight* magazine wounded or injured on active service P/O. N. E. Berrington-Pickett (42388).
29. Bob Marchant East Grinstead Museum 2024.
30. Ibid.
31. Bob Marchant East Grinstead Museum Bomber statistic 2022
32. The East Grinstead Museum data base of members identifies where the service trade of individuals is unknown.
33. R Davies and J. Hunter, 'A Recovery Ward: Its Planning and Use', *The Lancet*, 1952, pp. 865–8.
34. Royal College of Surgeons of England rcs: E005955.
35. 'Bill the Gardner', *The Guinea Pig*, 1944, p. 12.
36. 'Pigs on parade', *The Guinea Pig*, 1949, p. 20.
37. East Grinstead Museum data base and Guinea Pig Club memorial board.
38. The Guinea Pig Newsletter, distributed in 1944.
39. Edward Warburg, member of the Hamburg banking family, patron of the arts, former head of public relations at the Metropolitan Museum, New York. www.theartnewspaper.com

Chapter 2: The Queen Victoria Hospital

1. Harold Gillies, FRCS (1882–1960) considered to be the developer of modern plastic surgery, cousin of Archibald McIndoe. William Kelsey Fry (1889–1963) a dental surgeon of oral and maxillofacial surgery. Warwick James (1874–1965) dental surgeon.
2. 'The Pea-Nut Corner', *Kent & Sussex Courier*, 1939.
3. in October 1945, Mrs. Margaret Biddle, wife of an American Ambassador in Europe, purchased Saint Hill Estate. She commissioned a mural for the Manor ballroom undertaken by artist John Spencer Churchill, nephew of Sir Winston Churchill.
4. Bob Marchant, East Grinstead Museum.
5. *British Journal of Plastic Surgery* (1988), p. 423.
6. British Association of Plastic Reconstructive and Aesthetic Surgeons. Bapras collection.
7. 'Alexander (Alister) Burns Wallace FRCS (1906-1974)', *British Journal of Plastic Surgery*, 28 (2) (1975), pp. 149–50.
8. The title changed in 2006 to the *Journal of Plastic, Reconstructive & Aesthetic Surgery*.
9. *Journal of Plastic, Reconstructive & Aesthetic Surgery*, 16 September 2020. Murray C. Meikle, *Reconstructing Faces: The Art and Wartime Surgery of Gillies, Pickerill, McIndoe and Mowlem* (Otago University Press,) 2013, p.107
10. 'New Zealand plastic surgery story', *Australasian Journal of Plastic Surgery*, 2018.
11. *British Journal of Plastic Surgery* (1988), p. 423.
12. Ibid., p. 424.
13. Report, Fry to Hebb 1940, TNA: MH 76/116.
14. *Sussex Express* newspaper report.
15. *Sussex Express* newspaper report and *The Blitz Then and Now*, Vol. II, p. 139.
16. Reminiscences of 1938–1945 by Head Warden, T. P. Peters
17. www.roll-of-honour.com/Sussex/EastGrinsteadWWIICivilian.html
18. Leonard Mosley, *Faces from the Fire: The Biography of Sir Archibald McIndoe* (Weidenfeld and Nicolson, 19620, p. 163.

19. Ministry of Information Intelligence report No.145 15 July 1943 Covering period 6 to 13 July 1943.
20. Millar, 'Rooksdown House and the Rooksdown Club', p. 432.
21. Ibid., via Sid McQuillan Guinea Pig. The author identifies Nurse Mary as Mary Courtenay referenced by Richard Hillary in his book *The Last Enemy.*
22. M. Harrison, *Medicine and Victory: British Military Medicine in the Second World War* (Oxford University Press, 2004).
23. Archibald McIndoe, *Post-Graduate Medical Journal*, Vol. 19 No. 212 (1943), pp. 161–7.
24. Vitek Formanek.
25. *British Journal of Plastic Surgery* (1988), p. 425,
26. East Grinstead Museum data base and Bishops 1963 register.
27. E. J. Dennison, *A Cottage Hospital Grows Up: The Story of the Queen Victoria Hospital, East Grinstead* (Anthony Blond, 1963).
28. In June 1945 the Home Office gave permission for 1,000 children under 16 to be brought to England for recuperation and ultimate re-emigration overseas. The Committee for the Care of Children from Concentration Camps was established to monitor and care for the children. holocaustcentrenorth.org.uk
29. *West Sussex Gazette*, Thursday 10 July 1941.
30. P. Wilton, 'WW II Guinea Pigs played crucial role in refining plastic surgery in Canada', Canadian Medical Association Journal (1998); also quoted www.historic-uk.com/CultureUK/Guinea-Pig-Club.
31. The Military Museum, Calgary.
32. National Archives MH76/154.
33. AIR 29/764/9 Matlock Hospital formed September 1939, disbanded April 1945.
34. Squadron Leader S. C. Rexford-Welch (ed.), *The Royal Air Force Medical Services. Volume I: Administration* (HMSO, 1954), p. 308.
35. Bob Marchant, East Grinstead Museum, 2024.
36. Mosley, *Faces from the Fire*, p. 114.
37. Ibid., p. 108.
38. *Sussex Express* newspaper.
39. Mosley, *Faces from the Fire*, p. 117.
40. W. R. Feasby, B.A., M.D. (ed.), *Official History of the Canadian Medical Services 1939-1945* (1953 (Vol. 2) and 1956 (Vol. 1).
41. Ibid.
42. *The Guinea Pig*, July 1984, p. 7.
43. The Peanut Club lasted for many years beyond the war and funded gifts for children on the hospital's Burns Ward.
44. Lloyd's has a proud association with Admiral Lord Nelson going back to the Battle of the Nile in 1778 where a Lloyd's committee raised £38,000 to help the wounded and bereaved. www.lloyds.com
45. Mosley, *Faces from the Fire*, p. 168.
46. Mayhew, *Reconstruction of Warriors*, p. 195.
47. Mosley, *Faces from the Fire*, p. 162.
48. *British Journal of Plastic Surgery*, Vol 40 (January 1987), pp. 102–03.
49. *The Guinea Pig* (1981), Tribute p. 20.
50. Guinea Pig Sid McQuillan's memories to author.
51. 'Christmas greetings from a friend', *The Guinea Pig*, December 1949, p. 5.
52. Club newsletter April 1948, p. 30.

53. The East Grinstead Museum database indicates a significant number of entries where numbers of operations are unknown.
54. EGRTM 2773.523 – Photo of McIndoe, Guinea Pigs and nurses around piano, Christmas 1947, including Butler.
55. Air Vice Marshal Morley's McIndoe lecture, 1962.
56. *The East Grinstead Courier.*
57. Brian Cull, *Diver! Diver! Diver!: RAF and American Fighter Pilots Battle the V-1 Assault Over South-east England, 1944* (Grubb Street, 2008).
58. Donovan, 'As for the Canadians', p. 126.
59. W. R. Feasby, *Official History of the Canadian Medical Services 1939-1945, Volume II* (1953).
60. Ibid from notes by Bob Marchant.
61. Eric Taylor, *Women Who Went to War 1938-1946* (Robert Hale, 1988).
62. *The Guinea Pig* (1981), p. 26.
63. *Crawley and District Observer*, Saturday 19 January 1946.
64. The author considers this to be the foundation work which forms the major part of the East Grinstead Museum data base.
65. Guinea Pigs returning for further surgery were administered by Elsie Myson.
66. *The East Grinstead Society Bulletin*, No 126 (Autumn 2022).
67. *West Sussex Gazette*, Thursday 9 January 1947.
68. *Gloucester Citizen Newspaper*, 2 November 1949.
69. Charity Commission number 251271
70. Via son of Robert Chitham to Donald M. Norrie 2003 and *The Guinea Pig* (New Year 1994), pp. 5–6.
71. The British War Relief Society was a United States based humanitarian organisation dealing with the supply of non-military aid and financial aid to people in Great Britain during the Second World War. adp.library.ucsb.edu

Chapter 3: The Guinea Pigs in Wartime

1. *The Guinea Pig*, January 1999, p. 2. Post-war identity was George Glebocki.
2. P. D. Cornwell, *The Battle of France Then and Now*, p. 271.
3. Ibid., p. 356.
4. Patricia Lady Foley, wife of Herbert via D Erskin Hill, DNW Bolton St, Piccadilly.
5. *Nottingham Evening Post*, 2 October 1942.
6. 'Lost Weekend', *The Guinea Pig*, December 1954, p. 7: also P. Cornwell, *Battle of France Then and Now*, pp. 142, 213, 285 and 298.
7. Squadron Leader S. C. Rexford-Welch, *The Royal Air Force Medical Services*, Vol. 1, p. 460.
8. Ibid., The emergency medical services summary.
9, Rexford-Welch, *The Royal Air Force Medical Services*, Vol. 1, p. 313.
10. Ibid., p. 312.
11. Vanora, daughter of Sir Archie McIndoe, assisted in publishing Richard Pape's book *Boldness Be My Friend* (1953)
12. National Archives PoW repatriation reports. Sikorski Museum archives.
13. Josef Biel's correspondence was sold at auction. Joe Biel, Andre Brown, *The Guinea Pig*, July 1985, pp. 6–7. National Archives WO 416/29/302
14. Maurice Mounsdon's medals and memorabilia were sold at auction in 2022. Extracted detail of his injuries from catalogued source.
15. *The London Gazette* of 6 August 1940, No. 34915 awards of the Medal of the Military Division of the Most Excellent Order of the British Empire, for Gallantry.

16. The George Cross replaced the Empire Gallantry Medal. All holders of that award were instructed to exchange their medals, a substitution of awards unprecedented in the history of British decorations.
17. Christopher Shores, *Aces High Volume II*, p. 187.
18. *The London Gazette* of 4 June 1940 No. 34864.
19. AIR 81/300 Casualty File.
20. Steve Brew, *Blood Sweat and Courage: 41 Squadron* (2014). Operation tally quoted conflicts with museum data base.
21. 'Who's Who in the Guinea Pig Club', *The Guinea Pig*, Christmas 1953, p. 32.
22. Graham Warner, *The Bristol Blenheim* (Crecy Publishing, 2002), p. 306.
23. W. R. Chorley, *RAF Bomber Command Losses of the Second World War Vol 7: Operational Training Units 1940-1947* (2002).
24. Colin Pateman, *Goldfish Caterpillars and Guinea Pigs*, 24 June 1987, medals sold by the recipient's son at auction.
25. Jean-François Nothomb, alias 'Franco,' took over command of the escape line and led it from June 1943 until his arrest in January 1944. He was later awarded the DSO.
26. National archives WO 208/3313/1192 M.I.9/S/P/G (-)1192 evasion report.
27. www.iwm.org.uk/history/the-nation-at-a-standstill-shutdown-in-the-second-world-war
28. www.awm.gov.au/collection/C263314
29. East Grinstead Museum data erroneously indicates the name Henry Spooner 79122.
30. Flight Lieutenant Spooner 79133, *The London Gazette* of 6 June 1941, p. 3242.
31. Bob Marchant, East Grinstead Museum, 2024.
32. Michael Maton, *The Recipients of Foreign Awards* .
33. Norman Franks, *Fighter Command Losses* (1989), Vol 2, p. 34.
34. 'Men of The Battle of Britain, Kenneth Wynn and H.A.C. Bird-Wilson', *The Guinea Pig*, July 2001, p. 4.
35. Air Ministry Bulletin No. 8 of 27 February 1945
36. Maton, *The Recipients of Foreign Awards.* Award effective 6 February 1948 as per AFRO 81/48.
37. Donovan, 'As for the Canadians', p. 43.
38. Wellington R1641 300 Squadron. W. R. Chorley, *Bomber Command Losses 1941* (1998), p. 123.
39. *The Guinea Pig* New Year 1981- Flight wartime publication of rank.
40. East Grinstead Museum data records the forename as Henry. *The London Gazette* gives Harry.
41. The London Gazette of 31 October 1941
42. Of the 1,433 Hampdens built approximately half of the production run was lost on operations but a remarkable 458 aeroplanes were written off in accidents. Harry Moyle, *The Hampden File* (Tonbridge: Air Britain, 1989).
43. Air 2/4918 recommendation report, National Archives.
44. East Grinstead Museum database.
45. Beaufighter T5273 AIR 27/1508 National Archives.
46. The London Gazette of 20 May 1955, No. 2930,
47. 'Pity a Lonely Guinea Pig', *The Guinea Pig*, April 1948.
48. AIR2/8983 15 December 1943. *The London Gazette* of 11 February 1944.
49. Peter Smith, *Petlyakov PE2 "Peshka"* (Crowood Press, 2003), pp. 7–9.
50. David Charters, 'Gunshot wounds of both orbits', *The Lancet* January 1946
51. Club newsletter 1946
52. AIR 81/7892 National Archives – Spelling error of Baessonas.

53. 'SAS Tragedy at Sennecey-Le-Grand', *After the Battle* No. 120.
54. East Grinstead Museum via Bob Marchant.
55. Ibid.
56. 'Frostbite, how I became a Guinea Pig', *The Guinea Pig*, July 1986, p. 11.
57. 'Looking Back, Sid McQuillan', *The Guinea Pig*, Christmas 1966, pp. 23–5.
58. Colin Pateman, *Goldfish, Caterpillars & Guinea Pigs: Accounts of Pilots of Air Crews* (2012), Chapter 26, pp. 222–40.
59. The London Gazette of 17 December 1940, No. 35015,
60. D. Bruce, W. R. Chorley, and J. G. J. de Haan, 115 Squadron Roll of Honour.
61. 405 Squadron summary AIR 27/1787/15 formerly IIM/E405/1 Richard Turnbull R65168.
62. Donovan, 'As for the Canadians', p. 39.
63. Operations Record Books; Air Ministry Bulletin No.7328 dated 19/6/42 – No. 32 Air Ministry News Service.
64. 'A charming romance', *East Grinstead Gazette*, 24 March 1944.
65. National Archives casualty file (Air 81-9016) states it was a training flight.
66. The East Grinstead Museum data transposes his first names and reports a differing outcome for his admission.
67. Norman Franks, *Fighter Command Losses*, Vol 2, p. 37.
68. Air Ministry Bulletin 15584 dated 10 September 1944.
69. Australian War Memorial 65 4819 RAAF biographical file Stanley William Mitchell 422737.
70. *The Guinea Pig* first edition 1944 'Freddie is air sea rescued'.
71. Reid and Sigrist Ltd, managed by Major Reid and Frederick Sigrist, manufactured precision instruments, including those for aircraft. via *Graces guide to British Industry.*
72. Edward Bishop, *McIndoe's Army* (2001 edition), p. 107.
73. Kalarus was buried at St Cadwaladr Church Cemetery in Llangadwaladr Count Gwynedd (Wales)
74. 'Reminiscing', Christmas 1948 newsletter, p. 36.
75. Andrew Hendrie, *Canadian Squadrons in Coastal Command* (1997), p. 143.
76. Club newsletter August 1948, p. 23
77. Witold Krupa, *Flight Through the Storm* (Krakow 1992); listakrzystka.pl.pdf
78. 'Some of our Contributors', *The Guinea Pig*, April 1948, p. 42.
79. Colin Pateman, *Goldfish, Caterpillars & Guinea Pigs*, pp. 253–6.
80. Wellington Z1414 of 18 OTU was recalled to base but did not follow diversion instructions.
81. Wellington DV934 Operational training casualty. Caddel spelt Cadell on Guinea Pig Museum archives.
82. Colin Pateman, *Fuel Fire and Fear* (2018).
83. East Grinstead Museum data.
84. The National Archives WO 416, German Index cards of Second World War.
85. Bob Marchant, Guinea Pig Club membership secretary.
86. Ibid.
87. Donovan, 'As for the Canadians'.
88. On her retirement from the Queen Victoria Hospital in 1947 the Guinea Pigs paid tribute to her in their magazine, remembering her gentle and sure touch, and her humour and vivacious spirit.
89. Bob Marchant East Grinstead Museum extracted data.
90. www.flightglobal.com
91. East Grinstead Museum data.
92. www.telegraph.co.uk/news/obituaries/2460391/Bertram-Owen-Smith.html
93. National Archives AIR 81/18346.

94. Colin Hodgkinson, *Best Foot Forward: The Autobiography of the RAF's other Legless Fighter Pilot* (Barnsley, 2017), p. 63.
95. Mosley, *Faces from the Fire*.
96. 'Sam Gallop's Story', *The Guinea Pig*, New Year 1994, pp. 12–14.
97. Club newsletter December 1948, p. 40.
98. London Day article published 25 July 1946 unidentified newspaper.
99. November 16th 2010, Mr. Ed Melis gave a lecture at the National Liberation Museum 1944-1945 in Groesbeek. He said exaggerated bar talk and betrayal followed by a 'Van der Lubbe trial' would destroy the lives of these three young, skilled war pilots forever.
100. Leading Aircraftsman rank has only the rank of Aircraftsman below it, no flying aircrew held that low rank.
101. 'Guinea Pigs on Parade', *The Guinea Pig*, July 1982, pp. 33–4.
102. 'Brian Birks gives Gen on Round Pigs in Round Holes', club newsletter July 1947, p. 17.
103. East Grinstead Museum.
104. Official numbering system by Wing Commander Jim Routledge OMRS
105. Wellington HZ113 was based at the Operational Training Unit in Wellesbourne Warwickshire.
106. navymuseum.co.nz/explore/by-collections/oral-histories/quilter-lieutenant.
107. John Adam, *The Guinea Pig*, July 1987, p. 8.
108. Guinea Pig newsletter, December 1947, p. 24.
109. Commonwealth War Graves Commission. Squadron Leader Lane removed from Mandalay Cemetery to Taukkyan Cemetery. Special Forces Detached Burma. Headstone inscription from family. Of Blessed Memory. Roy Lane was from a family of three children, all sons who died flying in the Second World War.
110. Donovan, 'As for the Canadians', p. 161.
111. T9356 was delivered to the Netherlands 320 Squadron on 22 February 1941. Destroyed by fire 8 March 1941. AIR 81/5389 Flying Officer H. C. Prager (Netherlands), Pilot Officer F. Overeijnder (Netherlands), Corporal J. Zuurveld (Netherlands), Aircraftman A. Van Mastbergen (Netherlands), Aircraftman H. Jongman (Netherlands): injured; aircraft crashed on return from operational flight.
112. Henry Standen 1979.
113. AWM65 19 RAAF biographical files Adcock Ronald Sam 411846.
114. 'RAAF Pilot Wins DFC', *Sydney Morning Herald*, 11 July 1942, p. 11.
115. 'Guinea Pigs on Parade', *The Guinea Pig*, New Year 1981, p. 40.
116. The crash occurred when training with 1666 Heavy Conversion Unit, based at Wombleton in North Yorkshire.
117. Irish Military Archives, Dublin G2/X/1423 and ACF-S-259.

Chapter 4: A Legacy – The Guinea Pig Club and its Members after the War

1. Pelham Books Ltd, 1981.
2. www.rafmuseum.org.uk
3. East Grinstead Museum extracted data.
4. BBC Christmas broadcast transcribed from *East Grinstead Gazette* 29 December 1945
5. Robert Wright, *Night Fighter*.
6. Robert Wright, *Sholto Douglas. Years of Combat and Years of Command*. Robert Wright, *Dowding and the Battle of Britain*.
7. John Bird, *HMS Theseus: Five days in April 1946*.
8. *The Guinea Pig*, December 1956, p. 13.
9. Pigeons featured in Bomber Command magazine articles, such as in *Illustrated* on 21 November 1942.

10. 'Who's Who in the Guinea Pig Club', *The Guinea Pig*, August 1954, p. 28.
11. Tribute to Henry Standen, Club newsletter 1957, p. 42.
12. *The People* Newspaper 1 June 19 47.
13. Colin Pateman, *Goldfish, Caterpillars & Guinea Pigs*, Chapter 34, pp. 275–7.
14. 'Guinea Pig Goes East', *The Guinea Pig*, August 1948, pp. 13–14.
15. Ava Thompson is the Co-Trustee of the Ava Gardner Living Trust and the great-niece and namesake of Ava Gardner.
16. *The Guinea Pig*, December 1956, p. 36.
17. Club newsletter 1948, p. 29.
18. The Maestros published message 1948.
19. Maurice Buttler, *The Guinea Pig*, July 2002, p3
20. U.S. Edition September 27, 1948 Vol LII No.13.
21. Air Commodore Payne, *Air Dates*, 1957, p. 404.
22. *Flight* magazine wounded or injured P/O. N. E. Berrington-Pickett (42388). Club newsletter 1947, p. 3 quotes the spelling as A Benington-Pickett meeting McIndoe in Africa.
23. Parratt, Hugh Edmund (Oral history). 16279 Imperial War Museum.
24. 'On parade', Club newsletter 1950, p. 30.
25. Pre-decimalisation figure shown. On 1 February1971 one shilling 1/- became 5p therefore 8/6d equates to 43p
26. Steve Attwater, provision of service detail and image of his father.
27. Jimmy Edwards, *Six of the Best* (1984).
28. *The Guinea Pig*, Summer 1963, p. 12.
29. *West Sussex Gazette*, 10 October 1957
30. Annual General Meeting 28 September 1957 at the Queen Victoria Hospital.
31. Guinea Pig Dr. Sandy Saunders 2016.
32. *British Journal of Plastic Surgery* (1988), p. 428. The Bradshaw Lectures are given at the invitation of the Royal College of Physicians and the Royal College of Surgeons of England.
33. *The Guinea Pig*, August 1951, p. 9.
34. 'In memoriam', *The Guinea Pig*, Summer 1960, p. 45.
35. www.cwgc.org Cannock-chase-German-military-cemetery.
36. *The Guinea Pig*, Summer 1963, p. 19.
37. The brooches were commissioned by the Guinea Pig Club and cast by Klondyke Jewellers Limited. The master jeweller responsible was John Balcombe Meaden of Haywards Health, Sussex.
38. 'Topers Tale', *The Guinea Pig*, Summer 1963, p. 33.
39. Pre-decimalisation figure shown. On 15.2.1971 one shilling 1/- became 5p therefore 35/- equates to £1.80p
40. *London Gazette* issue/52767/supplement p8

Conclusion

1. Tom Dolezal, The Free Czechoslovak Air Force Associates Ltd.
2. Harold Frederick Avery. Canadian prisoner of war. Parachute escape when harness buckle smashed into his face. Rendered unconscious in fall 9.5.1942. Name mentioned *in Guinea Pig* Magazine. Repatriation facial repair of unknown detail. AIR81/14201.
3. Hans Raymond Anderson was admitted to the Queen Victoria Hospital on 2 September 1945.